Praise for
Running Doc's
to Healthy Eating

"Running Doc is back with his thoughts on nutrition and healthy eating. As one who has broken bread with him many times, I can testify he knows his way around good food. I highly recommend this book, which gives readers a simple approach to fuel their athletic performance, whether they are eating at home or on the go."

—**Steve Van Camp, MD,** cardiologist, past president
of the American College of Sports Medicine

"Dr. Maharam has been advising runners on how to stay healthy for over forty years. His latest book offers nutritional advice to fuel performance and prevent injuries. It should be on every runner's bookshelf."

—**John E. McNerney, DPM,** former team podiatrist,
New Jersey Nets and New York Giants

"I have known the Running Doc for many years. He is a complete sports physician, taking care of sports injuries, health, and wellness conditioning. With this book, he talks to you in a simple, easy to understand manner so you can eat healthy and perform better."

—**Rod Dixon,** four-time Olympian, Olympic medalist;
two-time World Cross-Country medalist;
New York City Marathon champion

"Without doubt, the Running Doc has written a gem here—with simple solutions and sound advice, the book makes it easy to be healthy and vibrant again."

—**Douglas S. Kalman PhD, RD,** adjunct professor,
Sports Nutrition, Nova Southeastern University

"Sports nutrition is as vital a part to a runner's success as is proper training. Dr. Maharam covers all the mile markers in *Running Doc's Guide to Healthy Eating*. A must-read for runners of all levels."

—**Andrea Chernus, RD, CDE, CSSD,** registered dietitian, certified specialist in sports dietetics

"I have known Dr. Maharam since our early days in New York City and watched as he built a thriving practice. Runners lined his waiting room because, as a primary care sports medicine doctor, he was able to help them feel better and perform better. Reading this book, you will feel as if the Running Doc is talking directly to you, guiding you to better food choices every step of the way."

—**Heidi Skolnik, MS, CDN, FACSM,** sports nutritionist to pro teams, marathoners, and performing artists

"Athletic performance is as much about your input as it is about your output. Dr. Maharam is to be commended for recognizing this with *Running Doc's Guide to Healthy Eating*."

—**Alexis Colvin, MD,** associate professor, Department of Orthopaedic Surgery, Icahn School of Medicine at Mount Sinai; team physician, U.S. Fed Cup team; chief medical officer, U.S. Open

RUNNING DOC'S™ GUIDE TO HEALTHY EATING

The Revolutionary 4-WEEK Program to Boost Your Athletic Performance, Everyday Activities, and Weight Loss

LEWIS G. MAHARAM, MD, FACSM

with Mark L. Fuerst

Foreword by Olympic runner Meb Keflezighi, Olympic silver medalist,
New York City and Boston Marathon champion

Health Communications, Inc.
Boca Raton, Florida

www.hcibooks.com

**Library of Congress Cataloging-in-Publication Data
is available through the Library of Congress**

© 2020 Lewis Maharam, MD, FACSM

ISBN-13: 978-0-7573-2204-4 (Paperback)
ISBN-10: 0-7573-2204-2 (Paperback)
ISBN-13: 978-0-7573-2205-1 (ePub)
ISBN-10: 0-7573-2205-0 (ePub)

Publisher: Health Communications, Inc.
        1700 NW 2nd Avenue
        Boca Raton, FL 33432-1653

Cover design by Larissa Hise Henoch
Interior design and formatting by Lawna Patterson Oldfield

To Welabucs…
Who knew…

CONTENTS

FOREWORD

*E*ven though I no longer run professionally—the 2017 New York City Marathon was my last competitive race—I still love to run, and I have stayed in a position to guide and inspire others to keep running.

I hope you use this book to become inspired to run or play your chosen sport and do your best. You are what you put in your system. This book can show you how to eat the best foods in an innovative way. As Dr. Maharam notes, during training, try different types of nutrition to see what works for you. And as he states, you need to hydrate weeks and months ahead, not just the day before a race.

This book also explains how to eat before and after a big event. Typically, before a long race, I would eat a lot more protein in the middle of the week, then as race day approached, I would eat more carbohydrates but not eliminate the protein. I love spaghetti. Or, I would eat rice or whole-wheat pasta as the main part of my dinner, with chicken or fish plus some green vegetables. You have to be careful of carbohydrate intake and not totally "carbo load."

I would also eat more salads and fruits, and graze throughout the day. For example, I like to have half a bagel toasted with almond butter or peanut butter with tea before I go for a morning run. I try to have five servings of fruits throughout the day to avoid hunger.

And I would make sure to hydrate. The best way to test your hydration is through the color of your urine, as Dr. Maharam describes. You want just a little color in your urine. I normally drink a lot of water. That way I would make sure I am hydrated before the gun goes off.

The first thing I do after a race is move around. Food is not yet immediately important. Within fifteen to twenty minutes of finishing, I have a recovery drink for quick energy right away. After a hard session or race, I like to use a UCAN shake to help me recover within a thirty-minute window. Then a few hours later, protein becomes very important. I might eat an omelet or steak. You can eat whatever protein you like.

Also include some fat in your diet after a long race. You deserve it! You need to eat some fat to build back the reserves you lost. I like chicken skin with my chicken. Avocado is always in my diet because it has good fats.

I have used cottage cheese and strawberry jam on a burrito if I get hungry at night after dinner. Or I use it as my dessert if I have a long run the next day.

When I run 130 miles a week in training, I demand a lot of my body. I make sure to eat a little more, as you will learn about in the Training Plate chapter of this book. I also get therapy regularly; for example, I go for a massage even when my muscles do not hurt badly because I want to tune up my body. "Prehab" is better than rehab.

If you run thirty miles a week, you still have to take care of your body. You may not run as many miles as me, but you can do a lot nutritionally to meet peak performance by eating and hydrating right. To hydrate, I recommend having a water bottle at your desk and sipping it throughout the day. You always have a choice. Squeeze in a run before work or at lunch. When you are motivated, you will have the discipline to eat and drink right.

I remember when I went to college in 1997, I ate as if every meal was my last. Growing up poor in Eritrea, there was not enough food on the table, so when I got to college I just ate as much as I could. One of my college professors had us write down everything we ate and all the exercise we did. The professor told us we needed to eat right as well as get enough exercise. This turned on a light bulb for me, and my running performance improved.

My race weight ranges from 121 to 125 pounds. When I'm injured, it goes up to 135 to 138 pounds, and I know I have to restrict my sugar intake to keep the weight down. Once I'm back running, the mileage will help me maintain my weight.

If you are injured, be careful because food can become your comfort. Make sure you stay on the path to recovery, and you will bounce back. Eat right at the time you need to. When you run less, you should be more disciplined with your diet. Find what works for you. If you can't run, read a book during lunch time. Don't just eat junk food. Use your free time wisely.

I didn't make the U.S. Olympic marathon team for the 2008 Games and found out I had a pelvic stress fracture, which Dr. Maharam helped me get through. I had to become more disciplined with my eating. I knew if I ate one doughnut, I would think, *Oh, another doughnut won't hurt*. While I was injured, I did a lot of cross-training, including biking and jogging in water. When I worked out in a pool, I knew I would be hungry when I came out of the water. I had a banana or shake ready in my car so I didn't eat doughnuts or chips.

Read this book, and you will learn how to eat so that you don't crave junk food. You will make the adjustments you need in your nutrition. Dr. Maharam visually dissects the food on your plate for you and shows you how much of these foods should be on the plate. Then you experiment to make it right just for you. This is a great concept that I highly recommend.

In this book, you will also learn about making your food colorful. A variety of foods is important. You don't want to eat just carbohydrates or protein; you want a balance. I like to eat a balanced diet of a salad, pasta, and chicken for dinner. You may prefer other foods, maybe green vegetables over wild rice and shrimp. At breakfast before a workout, I like to eat peanut butter or almond butter on toast plus a handful of berries. It might be eggs on a whole-wheat muffin plus an orange for you.

Dr. Maharam is very smart about nutrition and sports medicine. Even though I live in California, I go to see him in New York because I trust him. We talk about the best foods to eat and how to train. From this book, you, too, can learn from him what to eat to meet your athletic goals.

—Meb Keflezighi, *winner of the New York City Marathon,*
the Boston Marathon, and an Olympic Medal
(2004 Olympic Silver Medalist in Marathon)

ACKNOWLEDGMENTS

Undertaking a book like this requires many thank-yous and much appreciation.

Thank you Linda Konner, our extraordinary agent, who not only kept this project on track but connected the dots to actually make it happen; to Mark Fuerst for his powerful words and guidance; and Christine Belleris and the team at HCI Books for all their hard work and expertise to turn this concept into a book!

My wonderful, loving wife, Amy, provided the environment to get this book done. Thanks to my kids, Eddy, Melanie, Harris, and Lizzy, and my granddaughters, Cora Joy and her sister Gemma Beatrice, for their love and support.

Educators, professors, and doctors helped provide the foundation to be a good doctor: Mrs. Vovis, Dr. Majumdar, Dr. Doehler, Dr. Peace, Dr. J. Willis Hurst, Dr. H. Kenneth Walker, Dr. Corey Slovis, Dr. John McNerney, Dr. Allan Levy, Dr. Steve Van Camp, Dr. Ron Grelsamer, Dr. Evan Flatow, Fred Lebow, Tracy Sundlun, Allan Steinfeld, and Dr. Andres and Yolanda Rodriquez.

And to all of my patients: I learned early on that listening to my patients made me a better doctor. Thank you for your insights and stories.

—*Lewis G. Maharam MD, FACSM*

I would like to acknowledge the love and support of my family, Margie, Ben, and Sarah, through the long hours of writing and editing; the continuing love of my mother, Peppy; the camaraderie, brainstorming, and encouragement of the writers in the Brooklyn Brown Bag Lunch Group; and the lucid discussions with Dr. Maharam about nutrition and sports medicine that led to this book.

—*Mark L. Fuerst*

INTRODUCTION
From Food Pyramids to Fueling Plates

*T*hey call me Running Doc. The name fits because as a sports-medicine specialist, I see active patients and those who want to be active, and that usually involves running. When you think about it, most active sports involve running: tennis, soccer, basketball, baseball/softball, lacrosse, touch football, as well as triathlon.

As chairman of the International Marathon Medical Directors Association, I'm known by everyone in the running community, from professional racers to everyday exercisers. Of all my accomplishments, however, and what I'm proudest of, is the praise I get from my patients. As elite marathoner and Olympic medalist Meb Keflezighi says, "When runners get hurt, they fly to Dr. Maharam!"

If you're like me, when you drive into a gas station and pull up to the tank, you know that there's gasoline and diesel. I know I want gasoline. And then there are three different numbers, which I know stands for the amount of octane in the gasoline. It turns out that a company like Sunoco produces twenty-seven different blends of gasoline for different regions of the country, based on the climate, environment, and temperature. Some of these blends might contain an anti-icing component for the northern states, so the gasoline doesn't freeze in the engine. Some components for the South prevent algae from growing in gas tanks during hot summer months.

All of this got me thinking about how the blends of gasoline are similar to the diets of my patients. Carbohydrates are to the human body what oxygen is to the race car engine—it's what gets you to move. The higher the octane, the more power you get; the more carbohydrates you have in your body, the longer and harder you can go. The additives in gasoline are like a runner's use of vitamins, antioxidants, and supplements. But it's the carbohydrates that give you the "pop."

You've probably heard this before: Food is your fuel. But if we continue the analogy to a race car, what types of food allow you to increase your horsepower? What combination of foods allows your body to run at a higher rpm without overheating? That's what you'll find out in this book.

You can maximize your performance and speed by eating the correct amount of carbohydrates, protein, and fat. If you overdo one or don't have enough of the other, your performance and speed will suffer. Just as if you put something too thick in your gas tank, like sugar, or too thin, like water, your car won't run at all. The question, then, becomes: How much of each type of fuel does an exerciser need and at what time? Because just as all fuels are not the same, not all carbohydrates, proteins, and fats are the same.

The Old Food Pyramid

Chances are someone taught you about the U.S. Department of Agriculture food pyramid while you were growing up. The original 1992 Food Guide Pyramid had the "Breads, Cereal, Rice & Pasta

Group" on the bottom (six to eleven servings), working your way up through roughly three to five servings of the "Vegetable Group," the "Fruit Group," the "Milk, Yogurt & Cheese Group," and the "Meat, Poultry, Fish, Dry Beans & Nuts Group" all the way to the "Fats, Oils & Sweets," which come attached with the warning to use sparingly.

Now, let me ask you: Do you ever think about this when you are eating? Has this helped your understanding of the food groups? And what exactly is the size of a serving? The old food pyramid is nearly useless, yet it has influenced our perceptions of what constitutes a healthy diet, even subconsciously. You may subtly have these ideas that you were taught as a child and not even know it.

Then, in 2005, the USDA updated the old food pyramid and came out with the MyPyramid Food Guidance System, a new food pyramid. The ideas are spot on in a lot of places. They put an actual limit on sugar (10 percent of your daily calories), and they separated fats into "good" (saturated) and "bad" (unsaturated). But some of the same problems are still there. For example, there are too many different groups, and it's too hard to keep track of the arrangements within those groups. And these groups don't make sense in terms of how they are divided. A carbohydrate like French bread with a sky-high number of 95 on the glycemic index is lumped with whole-wheat spaghetti with a glycemic index of 37. This is just bad science.

What is the glycemic index? The glycemic index is a way to tell slower-acting "good carbohydrates" from the fast-acting "bad carbohydrates." You can use it to fine-tune your carbohydrate counting and help keep your blood sugar steady. In high-glycemic, fast-acting foods, sugars are used immediately and are readily available to your body—for example, fresh oranges, candy, and sports drinks. Low-glycemic or slow-acting carbohydrate foods, such as bread and pasta, are converted to simple sugars to be used later by your body.

Also, what is a "serving"? Let's take fruit, for example. Is a serving equal to one whole medium fruit? Is it one-quarter cup of dried fruit, a half-cup of canned fruit, or three-quarters of a cup of fruit juice? Actually, it is all of these in the new food pyramid! Now, how will you ever remember that?

The most important objection I have to this way of keeping track of our eating habits, and making changes within those habits, is that we don't eat our meals out of a pyramid. We eat them on a *plate*. And that is what this book will focus on. I will present you with a far simpler image—Fueling Plates—to begin exploring how to fuel your body optimally.

MyPlate Versus Fueling Plates

In 2011, the USDA introduced the MyPlate Plan as part of another update of food guidelines. This program showed a plate divided into four segments—fruits, vegetables, grains, and proteins—to try to grab consumers' attention with a new visual cue. It is not intended to provide specific messages, but rather as a reminder for healthy eating.

MyPlate is on the opposite end of the spectrum as prepackaged food plans, like Nutrisystem. In MyPlate, you add up the total number of calories and fat grams you eat; in Nutrisystem, someone has figured that out for you and provides you with a tray of food that's your dinner.

The MyPlate Plan is comparable to my Healthy Plate, but it doesn't go far enough. MyPlate has all the components of healthy eating, but it's too complicated to follow. In contrast, the Fueling

Plates program takes away all the calculations and has all the nutritional values of MyPlate. I have synthesized this information so that you get all the health benefits without having to do any math.

Another distinction is that there is no adjustment in the MyPlates program based on your fueling needs. Just as gas needs to be adjusted for climate, food intake needs adjustment, depending on whether you're going for a quick run or spending a few hours in one physical activity.

Also, choosing foods with MyPlate is easier to do in the house than in a restaurant. You can pick what foods you want to eat at home, weigh them, and calculate calories with MyPlate. It takes a good amount of time to do that in a restaurant. The beauty of the Fueling Plates program is its simplicity. You don't have to calculate how much you need to eat every day. This is easy to do all the time, and you can use it forever.

Using Fueling Plates, you will learn to divide your plate into quadrants: in the bottom right, fast-acting carbohydrates; in the bottom left, slow-acting carbohydrates; in the top right, protein; and in the top left, fats and anything else that you don't know what it is. I say that last part because a lot of times when you eat out, you will be served something, and it's like you are in an episode of the cooking show *Chopped*, where the contestants get something in their basket and they have no idea if it is a vegetable, a protein, or really what it is.

I'm going to tell you what I tell my professional athletes: Never consume anything without knowing exactly what it is. That includes performance-enhancing drugs and pills, of course, but also goes for your food. If you're looking at something and you can't decide what category it is, don't eat it! Or at least move it to that top left quarter, where how much of it you consume will be extremely limited.

Why Chefs Hate Me

Eating out is when most people have a difficult time figuring out what to eat—until now! I have friends who are chefs at restaurants, and they hate when the food comes and I take the gorgeous presentation they have worked so hard on and totally deconstruct it. That is what I will show you to do in this book: to divide your restaurant food on your plate into four quadrants, so that it looks like a child playing with food. We are going to take off the gravy and put it in the top left corner, which is going to be your fats. We'll put all your carbohydrates into the bottom part of the plate, splitting that up into fast-acting carbohydrates and slow-acting carbohydrates. And we'll put the protein in the top right corner.

This simple technique allows you, at a glance, to see there's too much fat here, or there's too much protein compared to carbohydrate. If you have ever been to New York City's famous Peter Luger Steak House, you know that the huge, delicious cut of meat you get will in no way fit into the top right of your plate. So, what to do? Cut the steak so it fits into that quadrant of the plate—and take the rest home!

And now you can easily figure out your ideal portion sizes. Portion size is another area where many nutrition books run amok. The Institute of Medicine, for example, recommends different allowances of protein and carbohydrates for runners: 56 grams per day for men and 46 grams for women. (Pregnant and nursing women need at least 71 grams of protein each day.) So, how do you figure that out? Are you going to carry around a little scale with you and weigh your food? No, but all of my patients complain that this is why nutrition books throw them for a loop. "Doc, it's all in grams!"

they say. Well, former president Jimmy Carter failed in his attempt to change us to the metric system, and neither these books nor I are going to be able to do that either.

The ease of portioning is what makes moving from food pyramids to Fueling Plates so beautiful. This book will show you how to figure out your basic metabolic profile by a simple self-assessment. Then you will know not only how much of your plate the protein should take up versus fat versus carbohydrates, but how high you should pile your food, based on both your body type and how often during the day you like to eat. With this understanding, you can build the perfect plate for you at different important junctures. Say you are looking to improve your tennis game, or play three sets on both Saturday and Sunday. You can shift your Fueling Plate into training mode, moving from the Healthy Plate to the Training Plate.

I provide specific Fueling Plate information for anyone interested in fueling for performance, from someone who was invited to run a 5K charity event, to a weekend pick-up basketball or soccer player, to the jogger who runs a few miles several times a week. I also have obtained recipes from high-profile chefs from restaurants I frequent, and show you how to move the foods around in each recipe for the Fueling Plates program.

Are you ready to learn an approach to nutrition that will stick with you for life, rather than a quick-fix approach that will be a constant battle to maintain? I'll bet you are. So let's dig into the Fueling Plates program that will teach you how much to eat and what types of foods to eat and how much liquid to drink to perform your best.

PART ONE

Sports Nutrition 101

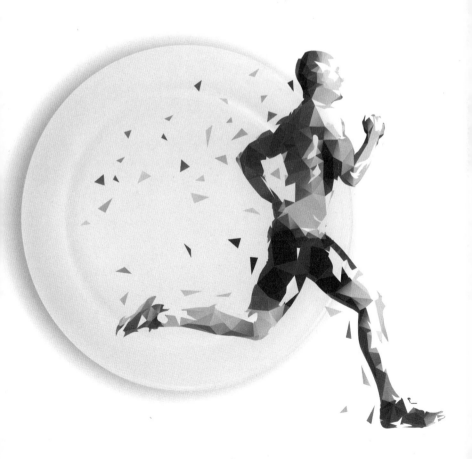

CHAPTER 1

The Only Three Food Groups You Need to Worry About

Jennifer, a thirty-two-year-old high school chemistry teacher, has run one marathon a year for the last seven years. "I plan on increasing my training this year so that I can run more races. I have been reading lots of nutrition information so that I can maximize my fueling. The American Heart Association recommends 15 to 25 percent daily calories should come from fats," said Jennifer. "Can that be right? I thought fats are bad for you."

When Jennifer came to see me, asking for nutritional advice, I told her that, yes, some fats are good in a runner's diet as an extra source of fuel. But picking the right type of fat is important to maintain a healthy lifestyle. We discussed what foods she eats, and I showed her how to use the Training Plate to prepare for races.

*T*he only three food groups you need to worry about are carbohydrates, fats, and proteins. Yes, there are other factors to consider for nutrition, and this book is not so simple that we are intentionally leaving out those other factors. It's just that you really only need to focus on these three food groups to be healthy.

When my patients, like Jennifer, ask me for nutritional advice, they often say they have read books that are too complicated and they can't follow the advice, or they don't want to spend so much time going through the book's program. I have read nutrition books myself and found that in order to live a healthy life and fuel yourself properly when you are active, you do not need to worry about the minor points. You need the big picture. If you do that right, you will be eating healthy food and need not worry about learning all the details found in nutrition books.

The first and main concept of Fueling Plates is it's important to know what carbohydrates, fats, and protein are. That means I want you to get away from nutritional chemical equations or learning about the amount of grams or calories in the foods you eat. Most complex diets are not so simple and easy to follow in your everyday life. They just complicate the matter of food choice. You will not find how many calories are in foods or how much energy leads to the breakdown of chemicals in this book.

Carbohydrates, fats, and proteins all deliver energy. The one thing you need to know is: how fast can I get at the energy? For the technically inclined, the fastest way to get energy is through glycolysis, or the breakdown of carbohydrates. As the sugar breaks down, it makes more adenosine triphosphate (ATP), the energy-carrying molecule found in the cells of all living things. ATP captures chemical energy obtained from the breakdown of food molecules and releases it to fuel other cellular processes. When the body's cells need energy, they convert energy from the storage molecules—carbohydrates, protein, and fats—into ATP. ATP then serves as a shuttle, delivering energy to places within the cell where energy-consuming activities are taking place.

Knowing how the body makes energy doesn't make you a smarter eater. Most importantly, you need to know that fast-acting carbohydrates, like simple sugars, break down into carbon dioxide and water. These fast-acting carbohydrates provide quick energy. The body uses fast-acting carbohydrates right away. Slow-acting carbohydrates, which are composed of more complex carbohydrates, take a longer time to make energy.

When your body lacks carbohydrates, it uses protein as an energy source. This source of energy is much slower than using carbohydrates. Protein is broken down into amino acids and is converted to acetylcholine and ketones. It takes longer to convert to amino acids, which are used to repair or replenish muscles, ligaments, and other tissues to allow you to do normal, everyday activities. These amino acids, in effect, rejuvenate your body.

Amino acids contain nitrogen. Even after the protein is digested into amino acids, the body must go through more steps to remove the nitrogen. This is why it takes longer to get energy from proteins than carbohydrates. Protein has other jobs that take priority over energy, such as building muscles and helping muscles work and the structures that support muscles (ligaments, tendons) to move.

Fats are the slowest energy producers. Fat is broken down into fatty acids. The body takes much more time to break down fatty acids to produce energy. That's why your body only uses fat when it has a desperate need for energy. Think about it: you can't sprint if you look like Jabba the Hutt. You need to find your ideal body weight with the help of your doctor. The Fueling Plates program can help you with that as well.

Calories are used to quantify energy. For every gram of carbohydrate or every gram of protein you eat, you get four calories of energy. Fats deliver nine calories per gram. Extra calories from food are stored in fat because it's the most concentrated source of energy. When your body needs energy, it first uses sugar from carbohydrates, then amino acids from protein, and finally fatty acids from fats. That's why your sweat smells like ammonia after a hard workout—your body has used fat that breaks down into fatty acids and ketones, a type of acid.

Ketones are chemicals made in your liver. You produce them when you don't have enough insulin in your body to turn sugar into energy. You need another source, so your body uses fat instead. Your liver turns this fat into ketones and sends them into your bloodstream.

"Good" Versus "Bad" Fats

As mentioned above, fats are used in the body as a storage form of energy. When you use up your carbohydrates, the fat that was stored is broken down into energy. Fats may be less efficient than carbohydrates as fuel, but they still provide an added bonus when you participate in a long-distance or endurance event.

There are four types of fats: two are "good" and two are "bad." The so-called bad fats are trans fats and saturated fats. Most trans fats are artificially produced by a process called partial hydrogenation. This process converts liquid oil into a solid. Saturated fats are typically solid at room temperature and can be found in meat.

The so-called bad fats have been shown to lower "good" high-density lipoprotein (HDL) cholesterol, raise "bad" low-density lipoprotein (LDL) cholesterol, and increase heart disease and stroke risks. You will find more information on cholesterol in Chapter 3. Try to avoid trans and saturated fats, which are found in meats, stick margarines and shortenings, butter, donuts, pie crusts, biscuits, french fries, and pizza dough.

It's important to note that these bad fats *can still be present* in foods even though the nutrition facts panel on prepared foods may claim 0 grams of trans fat. This is because the current regulations allow less than 0.5 grams of trans fat per serving. Smart athletes can find these hidden trans fats by reading the ingredients list and looking for partially hydrogenated oil. The American Heart Association recommends less than 1 percent of daily calories from trans fats and less than 7 percent from saturated fats.

"Good" fats are monounsaturated fats (omega-9) and polyunsaturated fats (omega-3). Monounsaturated and polyunsaturated fats are liquid at room temperature. These good fats are healthy and, yes, the American Heart Association recommends 15 to 25 percent of daily calories from this group of good fats. Good fats have been shown to decrease the risk of heart disease and stroke, reduce risk of diabetes, help maintain a healthy immune system, improve cholesterol profiles, improve vitamin absorption, and help nerve activity.

You can find these good fats in vegetable oils such as corn, canola, and sunflower oils. Other sources include but are not limited to nuts and seeds (walnuts and sunflower, for example); fatty fishes like herring, salmon, trout, and mackerel; avocado; eggs (the whole egg, not just the whites); poultry (chicken and turkey); dark chocolate; and coconut.

Not all fats are bad for you. If you routinely eat the good fats, in small quantities, you will add fuel to feel stronger in your chosen sport.

Top Ten Healthy Carbohydrate, Protein, and Fat-Rich Foods

I have compiled a few lists of healthy slow-acting and fast-acting carbohydrate foods, including slow-acting carbohydrate vegetables high in nutrients, protein-rich foods, and foods with healthy fat sources. Put these foods on your Fueling Plates for the best, healthiest way to provide your body the energy it needs.

Ten Slow-Acting Carbohydrate Foods

1. Oatmeal (old-fashioned or steel cut)
2. Brown rice
3. Sweet potatoes
4. White potatoes with skin
5. 100 percent whole-wheat bread
6. 100 percent whole-wheat pasta
7. Beans and lentils
8. Couscous
9. Butternut squash
10. Fresh beets

Ten Slow-Acting Carbohydrate Vegetables High in Nutrients

1. Asparagus
2. Salad greens
3. Tomatoes
4. Bell peppers (all colors)
5. Onions
6. Carrots
7. Cucumbers

8. Zucchini
9. Broccoli
10. Cauliflower

Ten Fast-Acting Carbohydrate Options

1. Banana (half)
2. Fruit juice (usually ½ to ¾ cup, or 4–6 ounces)
3. Glucose gel (one small tube is usually 15 g)
4. Orange juice (½ cup, or 4 ounces)
5. Raisins (2 tablespoons)
6. Nonfat milk (1 cup, or 8 ounces)
7. Soda with sugar (½ cup, or 4 ounces)
8. Sugar (1 tablespoon or 5 small sugar cubes)
9. Syrup (1 tablespoon)
10. Hard candies, jelly beans, and gumdrops

Ten Protein-Rich Foods

1. Eggs
2. Chicken breast
3. Salmon
4. Turkey breast
5. Canned tuna (solid white)
6. Nuts (walnuts, almonds, pecans)
7. Tofu
8. Flank steak (grass-fed beef)
9. Codfish
10. Greek yogurt

Ten Healthy Fat Sources

1. Almonds, walnuts
2. Olive oil
3. Avocado
4. Coconut oil
5. Salmon
6. Clarified butter
7. Ripe olives (all varieties)
8. Peanut oil
9. Pecans, cashews
10. Dark chocolate

Simple, Nutritious Diet

Weekend warriors need to have a simple, nutritious diet. Carbohydrates are considered "high-test" fuel. Different types of protein-containing or fat-filled foods are not as strong and powerful as carbohydrates to fuel an athlete's lifestyle. In general, I recommend you eat a diet with less sugar and one that is lower in cholesterol to prevent high lipid levels that can lead to plaque buildup in your heart and increase your risk of heart disease (see Chapter 3 for more on this).

Sometimes I have patients who tell me, "Carbohydrates are unhealthy. I'm going to eat less carbs and go on a keto diet." The problem with this idea is that you may not give yourself enough fuel or only provide "low-octane" fuel. You need to figure out the right amount of carbohydrates to put on your Fueling Plate to give yourself the energy you need for specific activities.

Why do I emphasize this? It's because you need different amounts of energy at different times. When you reach for a glass in your kitchen cabinet, your arms need a different amount of energy than when you are pumping your arms while running. If you are sprinting, you want more sugar on board from fast-acting carbohydrates and quick energy.

Superfoods

When you go shopping at the market, look for naturally brightly colored foods. Brightly colored foods contain more nutrients and therefore are more nutritious. The more color in the food, the more concentrated the nutrients.

"Superfoods" are foods that are thought to be nutritionally dense and therefore good for your health. But there are no set criteria for what makes a food a superfood. I think the term "superfood" is more of a marketing term for foods that have health benefits. Superfoods might be a good way for you to start thinking about healthy eating, but there are lots of healthy foods out there to explore, even if they aren't called "super." No dietitian or medical person will say superfoods are their own food group.

Below, I outline the most popular superfoods:

Blueberries often top the list of superfoods. They are rich in a multitude of vitamins and phytochemicals that come from the sun, as well as soluble fiber to help you move your bowels. *Phytochemicals* are compounds that are produced by plants ("phyto" means plant in Greek) that are believed to protect cells from damage. In young women, a diet rich in blueberries has been shown to reduce the risk of heart conditions. Blueberries usually take the top spot among superfoods, but that may be because they have been the most studied of the so-called superfoods. Other berries, such as strawberries, cranberries, and raspberries, also have high amounts of phytochemicals.

Kale is a dark, leafy green vegetable, like **spinach, Swiss chard,** and **mustard greens**. Kale is loaded with vitamins A, C, and K, as well as fiber and calcium. These vitamins help the body's metabolism at the microscopic level, and calcium helps build strong bones.

Sweet potatoes and **squash** are similar to leafy green vegetables in terms of the amount of fiber and vitamins A, C, and K.

Beans have multiple benefits. They provide a good source of low-fat protein and soluble fiber, which may help lower the risks of heart disease, and insoluble fiber, which adds bulk to the stool and appears to help food pass more quickly through the stomach and intestines. Beans contain loads of vitamins and minerals to help facilitate metabolic processes in the body, such as making energy to move muscles and making and repairing blood cells. The body's cells are constantly remodeling. This requires energy and vitamins and minerals to keep the cells working at optimal levels.

Whole grains have some valuable antioxidants not found in fruits and vegetables, as well as B vitamins, vitamin E, magnesium, iron, and fiber. Consuming foods rich in antioxidants may be good for your heart health and may also help to lower your risk of infections and some forms of cancer. Examples of whole grains include wheat, corn, rice, oats, barley, quinoa, sorghum, spelt, and rye.

Whole grains contain three parts: the bran, germ, and endosperm. The bran is the multi-layered outer skin that contains important antioxidants, B vitamins, and fiber. The germ (the embryo that can sprout into a new plant) contains many B vitamins, some protein, minerals, and healthy fats. The endosperm provides essential energy to the young plant to send roots down and sprouts up. The endosperm, the largest portion of the kernel, contains starchy carbohydrates, proteins, and small amounts of vitamins and minerals.

In contrast, "refined grains" are missing one or more of the three key parts. For example, white flour and white rice are refined grains because they both have had their bran and germ removed. Refined grains have about quarter less protein than whole grains and lose much of their nutrient value. Most of the grains around the world are eaten as refined grains. In response, many refined grains are now "enriched," meaning that a handful of missing nutrients are added back in. A better solution is simply to eat whole grains and garner the huge health advantages.

Medical evidence shows that whole grains reduce the risks of heart disease, stroke, cancer, diabetes, and obesity. Those who eat whole grains regularly have a lower risk of obesity, as measured by their body mass index and waist-to-hip ratios, and also have lower cholesterol levels.

Nuts and seeds are similar to whole grains in that they contain a high level of vitamins and minerals and are filling and nutritious. Many of my patients eat nuts and seeds to help them lose weight. They are healthy fats, and a handful of nuts and seeds can provide quick energy.

Fatty fish, such as **salmon, sardines,** and **mackerel,** are rich sources of omega-3 fatty acids, which are heart-healthy. Heart disease is mostly hereditary, even if you eat well, but it's always good to have fish in your diet a few times a week. I recommend swordfish, tile fish, smelt, and anchovies as well as the other fish mentioned above.

These foods are often considered superfoods. However, manufacturers rely heavily on marketing ploys, and lobbyists can shape public perception of products. Take the health benefits of macadamia nuts. A Hawaiian company lobbied the U.S. Food and Drug Administration (FDA) to make a health claim that macadamia nuts can reduce the risk of heart disease. The FDA released a carefully worded statement that 1.5 ounces of macadamia nuts per day as part of a low-fat, low-cholesterol diet could potentially reduce the risk of heart disease. Now consumers think macadamia nuts are a superfood that can help prevent heart disease.

Yes, macadamia nuts have good fat, and consuming macadamia nuts can be part of a good diet. They are delicious, and I enjoy them, in limited amounts, when I go to Hawaii. So you could include macadamia nuts as part of your Fueling Plate. But I wouldn't include macadamia nuts on a list of superfoods. If you eat macadamia nuts, you could miss out on another food that has just as good or better nutritional value.

Antioxidants

Another nutritional term that gets bandied about without much clarity is antioxidants. Most people don't really know what an antioxidant is.

Antioxidants are compounds produced in your body and found in foods. They help defend your cells from damage caused by potentially harmful molecules known as free radicals. When free radicals accumulate, they may cause a state known as *oxidative stress*. Oxidative stress may damage your DNA and other important structures in your cells. Chronic oxidative stress puts you at risk of chronic diseases, such as heart disease, type 2 diabetes, and cancer. Eating a diet rich in antioxidants can help increase the antioxidant levels in your blood and reduce the risk of these diseases.

"Anti" means against. Oxidants are formed as a normal product of aerobic metabolism, which is the way your body creates energy through the combustion of carbohydrates, proteins, and fats in the presence of oxygen. Antioxidants neutralize free radicals and prevent them from harming your body and causing premature aging and cancer, atherosclerosis, Alzheimer's disease, Parkinson's, and many other diseases.

Antioxidants are natural substances and can also be man-made. Whether you eat fresh vegetables or take antioxidants in a pill form, they may help your health. The typical antioxidants found in food include vitamins A, C, and E, beta carotene, lutein, lycopene, and selenium. When you think about eating healthily, eat fresh fruits and vegetables as a good source of antioxidants. Many clinical studies show that eating fresh fruits and vegetables lowers your risk of diseases, such as heart disease, diabetes, and high blood pressure. It's not entirely clear if it's the antioxidants or something else in these foods, but scientists believe it's the antioxidants. Frozen vegetables lose their strength and amount of antioxidants.

Some studies do link health risk to an excess of antioxidants. If you get too much beta carotene through foods or supplements, it appears to increase your risk of lung cancer if you smoke cigarettes. Also, high doses of vitamin E have been shown to increase the risk of one type of stroke and prostate cancer. If you take any antioxidant supplements, please discuss this with your doctor, that is, which ones you take and how much of each one, to avoid interactions with prescription medications.

Be careful, from a marketing standpoint, of how much attention to pay to advertising about the advantages of antioxidants to prevent and slow damage to cells. Doctors hope that antioxidants do prevent chronic disease since this makes sense. Medical research is strong, but not yet reproducible, of antioxidants as free radical Pac-Men that gobble up cells and make you healthier.

We know that eating fruits and vegetables will make you healthier. I suggest you stay with real healthy foods rather than taking antioxidant supplements. If you are thinking about consuming more antioxidants, eat more fruits and vegetables.

Where to Find Antioxidants in Foods

If you eat healthily, you're getting your antioxidants. There is no dietary allowance for antioxidants. It's enough to know that a high intake of plant-based foods is healthful. Here's a list of antioxidants and the common foods that contain them:

- Vitamin A in eggs, dairy, and liver.
- Vitamin C in fruits, especially berries.
- Beta carotene in peas, carrots, spinach, and mangoes.
  I especially love the Caribbean red mango, which has a lot of beta carotene.
- Vitamin E in vegetable oils, green leafy veggies, nuts, and seeds.
- Lycopene in red and pink fruits and vegetables, especially red Caribbean mango, tomatoes, and watermelon.

- Lutein in leafy green vegetables, papaya, corn, and oranges.
- Selenium in wheat, whole grains, rice, corn, nuts, eggs, and vegetables.

Other foods believed to be good sources of antioxidants include eggplant, black beans or kidney beans, green and black tea, red grapes, dark chocolate, blueberries, apples, broccoli, spinach, and lentils.

Be careful when you cook because you could increase or decrease the antioxidant levels in foods. If you cook down tomatoes, the amount of lycopene goes higher. But cooking cauliflower and zucchini reduces the antioxidant effect.

Fresh foods are always healthy. Think of yourself as a celebrity chef. What makes food so enticing on all of those cooking shows on television? It's all fresh. The fresher the foods you pick, the healthier they are. Just this thought will push you in the right direction to eat fresh fruits and vegetables, which is a good thing. My friend Thomas Keller, chef and proprietor of The French Laundry, Per Se, Bouchon, Bar Bouchon, Bouchon Bakery, and Ad Hoc, says active athletes who want to eat better should go to the market or store, pick out fresh fish, fruits, and vegetables, and cook them at home. That's the best way to know you have the freshest, and best, food on your plate.

Organic Foods

The term "organic" in foods comes from the way food is grown, handled, and processed. Produce must be grown without the use of most conventional pesticides, fertilizers that are not naturally made, sewage sludge, radiation, and genetically modified organisms. Animals cannot be given antibiotics or hormones.

Be aware that "organic" and "natural" are not interchangeable terms. In general, "natural" on a food label means that it has no artificial colors, flavors, or preservatives. It does not refer to the methods or materials used to produce the food ingredients. The USDA has guidelines on how organic foods are described on product labels:

- **100 percent organic.** This description is used on certified organic fruits, vegetables, eggs, meat, or other single-ingredient foods. It may also be used on multi-ingredient foods if all of the ingredients are certified organic, excluding salt and water. These may have a USDA seal.
- **Organic.** If a multi-ingredient food is labeled organic, at least 95 percent of the ingredients are certified organic, excluding salt and water. The nonorganic items must be from a USDA list of approved additional ingredients. These also may have a USDA seal.
- **Made with organic.** If a multi-ingredient product has at least 70 percent certified organic ingredients, it may have a "made with organic" ingredients label. The ingredient list must identify which ingredients are organic. These products may not carry a USDA seal.
- **Organic ingredients.** If less than 70 percent of a multi-ingredient product is certified organic, it may not be labeled as organic or carry a USDA seal. The ingredient list can indicate which ingredients are organic.

The idea behind organic food is that it's natural, and natural is better for the soil, environment, and your body. There is tons of research on organic foods not using certain pesticides and that's why they are healthier than conventional foods and also why the high cost of organic foods is worth it. However, the price of organics is higher than it should be.

Some of my patients are willing to pay as much as twice the price to get something organic. For example, at Walmart a can of organic pumpkin sells for 22 cents an ounce, which is twice as much as non-organic pumpkin at the same time of year in the same store. The USDA has found the costs of organic fruits and vegetables typically run more than 20 percent higher than conventional produce. Sometimes the difference is much higher, especially for organic milk and eggs.

A Stanford Medicine study compared the nutritional value of organic versus non-organic foods and found little difference between the two. Also, the amount of difference in taste between organic and conventional food is negligible. If you make the choice of organic foods for health, there may not be much difference. In reality, eating organic drives you toward eating fresh fruits and vegetables and raises your environmental consciousness. Both of these are good, so if you can afford it, go for organic foods.

The different pesticides in organic foods may not be significant enough for you to worry about. Organic farmers are not allowed to use synthetic fertilizers or pesticides, but they can apply ones made from natural ingredients, which can still be dangerous for your health.

When it comes to meat, organic beef, poultry, and pork may be free of synthetic pesticides and fertilizers, and antibiotics that are commonly given to animals on conventional farms. Regular use of antibiotics can lead to dangerous antibiotic-resistant bacteria. If you do buy conventional meat, trim off the fat and skin because they contain most of the pesticides.

The premise of this chapter is to keep it as simple as possible when choosing healthy foods. Many people who want to eat healthy or lose weight go to a packaged food company, like Jenny Craig, Nutrisystem, or South Beach Diet. If you want to eat healthily, and probably lose weight, you don't need to think so much. Just understand about these three food groups—carbohydrates, protein, and fats—where they come from and how to eat them. If possible, choose fresh fruits and vegetables, as well as fresh fish, chicken, and beef (but not every day), and fit them on your Fueling Plate.

I also want to emphasize that you want a healthy, varied diet. If you eat the same thing every day, you may miss out on essential vitamins and minerals. For example, if you ate exclusively green beans, you would not get the amount of vitamin C that's available if you also ate oranges. So eat both green beans and oranges. If you don't eat grains, you may not get enough vitamin B12. The idea is to not only know what type of foods to put on your Fueling Plate, but to put a variety of foods on the plate to get all the good nutrients you need.

Diet is a personal choice. We are all creatures of habit. My absolute favorite dish is cornflake chicken. I would choose it almost every day, but I know I need variety and can't eat chicken all the time. So I also eat shrimp, scallops, dover sole, along with vegetables, such as spinach, asparagus, beets, green beans, mixed-color carrots, potatoes and yams, and fruits including oranges, grapefruit, apples, melons of all kinds, berries, and pineapple.

So make sure you enjoy good, healthy foods, locally sourced if possible, now available in grocery stores, and look for foods with good, strong colors. With more variety in your diet, you will get the most benefit from eating their fuel and get your full complement of carbohydrates, fats, and proteins.

In the next chapter, I will tell you what to drink, how much, and when to drink before, during, and after a workout.

CHAPTER TWO

Hydration: What to Drink, When, and How Much

No discussion of sports nutrition is complete without delving into the topic of hydration. I will show you how to track your everyday fluid needs—what, when, and how much—before, during, and after exercise. I also describe the process by which sports drinks promote water absorption and bust the "sweat rate" myth (which states that you must replace the fluids you use during an event). We will also investigate the old wives' tale that everyone should drink eight glasses of water a day.

This chapter will discuss the dangers of over-hydration, along with how different variables such as temperature, humidity, and altitude can alter your hydration needs. And just as with food, I'll make hydration simple to understand, giving you an easy urine test to tell if you need to drink more or less (hint: aim for a lemonade-like color, as opposed to iced tea or water).

Hydration is important because all of our body mechanisms are based on fluids. Your body's fluids percentage is way higher than solids—estimates range from 60 percent up to 80 percent of your body is fluids. Every bodily system requires fluid for movement and flushing of toxins, as well as carrying nutrients to your cells and helping organs do their normal functions.

You need to replenish fluids so your body works at a pace it needs to be at its best. When you are dehydrated, your muscles work more slowly, and microscopic chemical reactions in your body are slowed down as well. Even mild dehydration can make you tired and feel as if you have less energy.

The Urine Test

The quickest and easiest way to know if you are properly hydrated is to look at your urine. If it looks like the color of iced tea, you need to drink more. If it looks like lemonade, you are well hydrated. If it's clear, you are drinking too much liquid.

You don't necessarily need to drink more before you get active. Definitely drink during activity and afterwards, if you're thirsty. Drinking more to get your urine into a clear state will not necessarily help and could harm you.

The urine test works so well because, like the Fueling Plates concept, it's simple. Your body has three possible colors of urine. That's exactly enough.

If you want to calculate your sweat rate before a road race, for example, here are the steps you would need to follow:

1. Weigh yourself nude before the race.
2. Run or walk at race pace for one hour. (One hour is recommended to get a reliable representation of the sweat rate expected in an endurance event.)

3. Track your fluid intake during the run or walk, measured in ounces.

4. Record your nude weight within an hour after the run/walk. Subtract from starting weight. Convert the difference in body weight to ounces.

5. To determine your hourly sweat rate, add to this value the volume of fluid consumed (from Step 3).

6. To determine how much to drink every fifteen minutes, divide the hourly sweat rate by four. This becomes the guideline for fluid intake every fifteen minutes of a run.

7. Note the environmental conditions on race day and repeat the measurements on another day when the environmental conditions are different. This will give you an idea of how different conditions affect your sweat rate.

No one says you have to drink as much as you sweat in order to perform at your best. The research shows there's a range you need to be within to get your best performance. You know the range by looking at your urine. So keep it simple! You do not need to chart your hydration status and sweat rate. Just check your urine.

Old Wives' Tale—Eight Glasses a Day

Everyone has heard the advice "drink eight eight-ounce glasses" of water a day. That equals about two liters of fluid a day. The Institute of Medicine has recommended that amount of fluid, as it is easy to remember, but there is no scientific evidence to back up that recommendation.

The old wives' tale of eight glasses, eight times a day does not work for everyone. Keeping up your body fluids is different for everyone, depending on your height and weight, total body surface area, metabolic rate, and sweat rate. Also, the weather and humidity are factors that change your fluid requirements. It's important for you to experiment to determine your fluid needs during training so you know what you need during an event. I always say that race day should be done exactly as you train. Do nothing new on race day!

Use your innate thirst mechanism to guide fluid consumption. This strategy should provide sufficient fluid to prevent excessive dehydration and limit drinking in excess.

Fitness and Vitamin Waters

My favorite drink if you're thirsty is plain old water, but fitness and vitamin waters have been heavily promoted to athletes. Fitness waters and vitamin waters are lightly flavored alternatives to plain water, sometimes colored and often enhanced with electrolytes, sugar, vitamins, and minerals. They were created in response to research showing that many exercisers don't drink enough fluids before, during, and after workouts. Companies reasoned that active people might be more likely to drink a flavored, colored beverage than plain water, resulting in better hydration.

Are fitness waters and vitamin waters better for you than plain water? The added electrolytes, sugar, vitamins, and minerals may help with post-exercise muscle soreness. Other than that, the main reason to choose flavored water is if you are more likely to drink it than plain water.

Fitness and vitamin waters are different from sports drinks. They contain only about ten calories per eight-ounce serving as compared to fifty or more calories per serving in a sports drink. Therefore, fitness and vitamin waters are not optimal for fuel replacement during a long workout or race or on a hot day when you lose electrolytes through sweat. Drink fitness or vitamin water when you would typically drink plain water, such as during a workout of less than a half-hour or a 5K to 10K race on a cool day. Stick to sports drinks when you need to rehydrate and refuel for performance during longer workouts (half-hour or more) and races, or on warm days when you will be sweating profusely.

Sports Drinks and Water Absorption

Do sports drinks promote water absorption? The answer is "Yes." The added sugar in sports drinks helps diffuse the water, salt, electrolytes, and minerals across cell membranes. This is what's known as an *active transport pump*. This cellular process is what makes sports drinks better than vitamin water if you want to get sugar across cell membranes for rapid energy. It's like a combination lock—the sugar, salt, and water all together turn the tumblers and get more sugar and water into your body's cells. A sports drink is designed to provide flavor, fluid, and electrolytes in an amount that can be absorbed rapidly without causing gut distress. Active individuals will have no trouble metabolizing the sugar found in sports drinks.

If sugar is an issue, for example, if you are diabetic, then during activity alternate a sports drink with water. There's no right mixture of sports drinks or water. I could tell you one way to use fluids, but it could be way too much or not enough for you. You need to use both sports drinks and water during practice, and check your urine to stay properly hydrated.

In general, sports drinks should be consumed along with water for runs that last more than ninety minutes. Drink about 16 ounces of water or sports drink the morning prior to your long run. During the run, drink no more than one cup (8 ounces) of fluid every twenty minutes while exercising. Be sure to stop for water or sports drink at fluid stations. (THIS DOES NOT MEAN EVERY STATION!)

For runs longer than ninety minutes, you must drink sports drinks. Drinking on the run requires careful planning of the route. Make sure you have enough water or sports drink available, and also stash the fluids if you do it on your own. Basically, you want to drink for thirst. Drink enough to get your urine to yellow, but not clear.

Hyponatremia

Susan, a fifty-six-year-old real estate agent, was playing in her club's tennis championship when she suddenly collapsed in the third set. "I started throwing up, I didn't know what day it was, and I blacked out. I ended up in the hospital," she said. "My husband, Frank, told the ER doctor that I had been drinking plenty of fluids because it was a hot day. I later remembered I had gone through three big bottles of sports drink."

The doctor confirmed his suspicion that Susan was hyponatremic by measuring the sodium level in her blood, which was extremely low. "I learned a hard lesson. Now I drink plenty of water before a match and drink just when I'm thirsty during change overs, and I alternate sports drinks with water," said Susan.

If you drink so much your urine is clear you are at risk for hyponatremia. Hyponatremia means a reduced concentration of sodium in the blood. If the sodium level falls below 129 mmol per liter, it creates, in mild cases, a general clouding of consciousness; you may feel your brain function slowing as if you were drunk. You may also be nauseous and vomit, and feel lightheaded and dizzy.

Drinking too much overwhelms the ability of the kidneys to excrete the excess water load. Sodium in the body becomes diluted, and this leads to swelling in cells, which can be life-threatening. The brain swells as the sodium level gets lower as a result from the general state of fluid overload.

In the most severe cases, hyponatremia can lead to unconsciousness, epileptic-like seizures, and possibly breathing problems or a heart attack. Fluid overload of the lungs may produce pulmonary edema that leads to shortness of breath and coughing up blood-stained sputum. During long races, I have seen runners with severe hyponatremia who have gross swelling of the hands and forearms.

How and why do you get hyponatremia? When you run or walk a long distance (10K or more), or play tennis or soccer for a long time, blood is shunted to the legs. That means less blood flow to the kidneys, which regulate salt. When blood is directed away, the kidneys' hormonal mechanism goes haywire, and salt regulatory hormones increase inappropriately. This causes the kidneys to concentrate your urine with salt and retain free water, even if you drink a salted drink or get intravenous fluid with salt.

Drinking too much fluid during prolonged exercise can lead to this dangerous condition. I usually see this condition in athletes who drink more than one cup (8 ounces) every twenty minutes. If you ran a marathon and stopped at every water station and drank just one cup of water, you would be hyponatremic by mile seventeen! As a result of overdrinking, you develop progressive fluid overload.

Who gets hyponatremia most commonly? First-time marathoners and participants in charity runs, who are usually first-timers, tend to be at risk. They fear they will become dehydrated in the heat and wrongly drink too much, not understanding the danger. They see everyone else drinking and want to drink also. Water stations are there in case you get thirsty, not because they want you to drink at every stop. I can't emphasize enough, *drink only when you're thirsty.*

Women are at much greater risk than men for reasons that sports scientists don't yet understand. I think it's purely a size effect; women are smaller and more likely to develop a fluid overload simply because it takes less fluid for smaller people to become overloaded. Alternatively, it's clear that a big part of the problem is the inability of the exerciser to excrete the excess fluid because of high levels of fluid-retaining hormones.

If you take non-steroidal anti-inflammatory drugs (NSAIDs) such as Advil, Aleve, Motrin, naproxen, ibuprofen, or aspirin, you are also at increased risk. These drugs work by blocking prostaglandins, a group of lipids made at sites of tissue damage or infection that are involved in dealing with injury and illness. By blocking prostaglandins, blood flow is decreased to the kidney, which sets up the cascade that increases fluid-retaining hormones.

It's not just marathoners who are at risk. Athletes who compete in triathlons, tennis and soccer players, canoe racers and swimmers, hikers, football players, and even yoga enthusiasts can succumb to hyponatremia. Athletes often are mistakenly advised to "push fluids" or drink more than their thirst dictates by, for example, drinking to a prescribed schedule. But excessive fluid intake does not prevent fatigue, muscle cramps, or heat stroke. Muscle cramps and heatstroke are not related to dehydration. You get heat stroke because you're producing too much heat.

Modest to moderate levels of dehydration are tolerable and pose little risk to otherwise healthy athletes. You can safely lose up to 3 percent of your body weight during a competition due to dehydration without loss of performance.

How can you make sure you are getting enough fluids, but not so much as to be at risk for hyponatremia? If you are drinking no more than one cup every twenty minutes, you will have enough fluids. The risk of dehydration, even in the heat, is far less than developing hyponatremia. Not drinking at every water station of a long race will prevent hyponatremia.

How can you spot hyponatremia in another athlete? Aside from some medical conditions that are usually well recognized, there are really few conditions specific to sport that cause an altered level of consciousness, nausea, vomiting, feeling light-headed and dizzy during or after prolonged exercise. These are exercise-associated collapse, dehydration, heat stroke, and hyponatremia.

Measuring body temperature is the first step to rule out hyponatremia. If the body temperature is above 102°F, the diagnosis is heatstroke. Place the athlete in or on ice to lower his or her body temperature. If the temperature is normal, then strongly consider the diagnosis of hyponatremia. The diagnosis can be confirmed by measuring the blood sodium content, obtaining a result below 129 mmol per liter. Medical doctors on the scene of a race are trained in evaluating these conditions and, if they suspect hyponatremia, will call for a transport.

What should be done for a stricken athlete? Giving the athlete one small salt packet under the tongue is a good start. The best treatment of the hyponatremia due to exercise is inactivity. Given time, the body will start to get rid of excess fluid by increasing urine production. Full correction of hyponatremia requires that the athlete gradually ingest some salt over the next ten to twelve hours.

Do not give any fluids to an athlete with an altered level of consciousness. First, determine whether the athlete may be suffering from hyponatremia. Mild levels of dehydration do not cause loss of consciousness. Giving fluid to hyponatremic athletes will, at best, worsen the condition and delay recovery. At worst, it may produce respiratory or cardiac arrest as a result of a sudden worsening of the brain swelling.

Anyone suspected of having hyponatremia should be transported to the hospital. At the hospital, doctors may choose to manage the condition by replacing the lost salt with a very concentrated (3 percent) salt solution—about three times higher than the concentration in normal saline solution—given intravenously at a very slow rate. This hypertonic saline solution can only be given in a hospital setting with proper monitoring.

To avoid hyponatremia during a long event, I recommend you follow these easy guidelines. Try these things on training runs beforehand to see how your body reacts:

- Follow the fluid recommendations and drink only when thirsty!
- Include pretzels, olives, or a salted bagel in your pre-event meal.
- Favor a sports drink that has some sodium in it over water, which has none.
- In the days before the event, add salt to your foods, provided that you don't have high blood pressure or your doctor has restricted your salt intake.
- Eat salted pretzels during the last half of the event.
- Do the salt! Carry two small salt packets with you (the kind found in fast-food restaurants). Before the event and again

during the last half of the event, consume a single packet under your tongue.

- After the event, drink a sports drink that has sodium in it and eat some pretzels, olives, or a salted bagel.
- Stop taking NSAIDs twenty-four hours before your event and do not start again until six hours afterward.

The risk of hyponatremia is so great that some marathon organizers have suggested reducing the number of water stations to five during a race. I do not believe that cutting down the number of water stations would work at major marathons. Everyone is an individual, and the event management attempts to create a safe environment for all. Where you get thirsty is individual. Having frequent fluid stations available gives everyone the option to drink when thirsty and not lapse into a "Where is the water?" panic. You should expect to see many fluid stations and then decide when to drink.

Dehydration is really not a serious concern at modern marathons. Only in the desert do we see dehydration that can't be corrected solely by drinking fluids.

Temperature, Humidity, and Altitude

The combination of high temperature and high humidity can make you sweat more. Your normal fluid replacement rate may need to be adjusted when you travel for vacation or a race because the climate and humidity are different from what you're used to. If you train in a different environment, sweat rates are only an estimate.

Your body is trained and acclimated to how much fluid it needs. If you travel, you will need to adjust your hydration needs, based on where you are. If you live in New Orleans and fly to Phoenix, your

hydration needs will be different than at home. At higher temperatures, your fluid intake will probably go up when you are active. If
possible, let your body acclimate to the new temperature for a few
days, if not a few weeks.

Higher humidity may make you sweat more. It's easier to sweat if
there is fluid in the air. So again, you may need more fluids. Similarly,
if you go to race at a high altitude, you will likely need more fluids.

If you go on vacation and plan to work out, your fluid needs
may change due to changes in heat, humidity, and altitude. After a
few hours of activity, look at your urine to see whether you need
to increase your fluid intake. Not everyone needs more fluid. Your
body metabolism may be so efficient that you don't need more. Just
know that a new climate may increase your needs, so please take a
look at your urine color. All you can do is monitor your own body.

Do icy, slushy drinks keep you cooler in hot weather? People
are always looking for new ways to keep cool during exercise and
one recent trend is drinking ice slushies (a mix of crushed ice and
water). Researchers have compared the amount of heat loss inside
the stomach during cycling and measured the differences in heat
loss from the skin because of altered sweating. It turns out those
who drank ice slushies had a sweat rate decrease so much that the
reduction in evaporation from the skin cancelled out the extra heat
loss in the stomach. In fact, overall internal plus external heat loss
was lower with an ice slushy drink. This and other studies suggest
that when you exercise in the heat, stick to drinking water (not ice)
at whatever temperature you prefer.

I participated in the development of a summary on fluids by
marathon medical directors around the world who came together
to discuss hydration for long-distance runners. For decades, runners

have complained that when they go to places with high temperatures, they use more fluid and needed guidelines. Here are the recommendations:

Most of Arizona is located in a desert, and for those traveling to those parts of the state to run a race, a unique drinking strategy is necessary to achieve optimum health on race day. If you do not have one week to acclimatize in Arizona's arid environment, it is recommended that, from the moment you arrive, you concentrate on optimally hydrating before race day. Liquid is lost in your breath and in sweat, and if you follow these directions, you will be healthy and perform your best.

Upon your arrival in Arizona, drink a sports drink with its added electrolytes until your urine appears to be a light lemonade color. Iced tea color is too concentrated; clear is too hydrated. Continue drinking sports drink in quantities that maintain this light lemonade color up until race morning.

On race day: DO NOT OVERDRINK! Hyponatremia (too low blood sodium/salt level) can occur while walking/running an endurance event if you drink too much. Drink no more than one cup (8 ounces) every twenty minutes during the race or as new medical research shows, you may drink enough to satisfy your thirst.

On race day bring two fast-food packets of salt. Eat one in the corral and the second one halfway through the event.

Do not take NSAIDs like Motrin, Aleve, or aspirin. They decrease blood flow to the kidneys and become an increased risk for getting hyponatremia. Tylenol (acetaminophen) is safe to take.

Do not take any pills or supplements that may cause dehydration. These include energy and diet pills, cold medicines, and anti-diarrhea products. Stay away from caffeine, which has dehydrating properties.

After the event, again check your urine color. Now you may have a sports drink with its added electrolytes until your urine is again light lemonade color. Once it is, you have normalized your hydration status and may eat and drink as you normally would.

The main point of this chapter is the very best way to determine your individual fluid needs is to monitor your urine. If your urine is clear, you are drinking too much and risking hyponatremia (low salt level in the blood). If your urine looks like lemonade, you are drinking the perfect amount for your individual needs. If your urine looks like iced tea, it is too concentrated, and you need to drink more.

The next chapter looks at how you can lower cholesterol with lifestyle changes.

CHAPTER THREE

Lowering Cholesterol with Lifestyle

Ann, an advertising executive, started running at age forty-five to stay alive. Her father, who didn't exercise at all, had died of a heart attack at age forty-five. "Since my father died of heart problems, I thought I should run to help keep down my cholesterol level, which my doctor said was high, over 200. I also started taking garlic pills to lower my 'bad' cholesterol number," said Ann.

Six months into her new regime Ann's cholesterol was still high. "I was upset. The running and garlic was not enough. My doctor prescribed a statin to help bring my cholesterol level down," she said. One month later, a follow-up check-up showed her cholesterol profile was excellent. Now age fifty-five, Ann has never had any heart problems and still runs three marathons a year. Because her age now adds to her heart disease risk factors, she is under the care of a cardiologist to monitor her health.

*I*f you have been putting in the miles to train for a long run like a marathon, you may be concerned about whether you are doing some good to your heart, especially when it comes to cholesterol levels. In 1991, I participated in a study on runners at the New York City Marathon that was subsequently presented at the American College of Sports Medicine Annual Meeting. The study suggested that when it comes to your total cholesterol count, not only is exercise good, but more exercise is better.

The news was in the "more." Although exercise has long been associated with good health, very little hard research had been done on the relationship between the amount of exercise and the degree of freedom from health risk factors, like high cholesterol levels. We tested highly conditioned athletes, such as those prepared to run a marathon in just a few days, and compared them to fit but less highly conditioned subjects, in this case, the people who accompanied the marathoners to the number pickup exhibit hall.

By race time, we had tested more than 2,100 runners and non-runners for total cholesterol. The runners were those going to the marathon starting line, and the non-runners were their friends and family—not necessarily a sedentary group to be sure, but they averaged a slower training pace and fewer weekly miles than did the runners.

In order to test thousands of subjects, we stuck with measuring total cholesterol rather than determining the more descriptive but time-consuming "good" high-density lipoprotein (HDL) cholesterol and "bad" low-density lipoprotein (LDL) cholesterol values. Even so, it was apparent that all our subjects were well under the typical 200-plus total cholesterol count found in the general population, and that the marathon runners had values lower still than their lesser-trained companions.

We were hardly surprised to find that older subjects—runners and non-runners alike—had higher cholesterol values than younger ones, and those who weighed more and were heavier for their heights (higher weight/height ratios) also tended to have higher cholesterol levels. The big exception was among the women pre-pared to run the marathon. For all practical purposes, their choles-terol levels had no statistical link to either their weights or their weight/height ratios. Older women did have reliably higher values, but poundage apparently had nothing to do with it. There are lots of possibilities for our finding, including the fact that we did not separate out pre- and post-menopausal women. Estrogen is thought to have a protective role when it comes to cholesterol.

But one recommendation is incontrovertible from our study: keep exercising. Healthier low total cholesterol profiles are unequiv-ocally associated with some of the healthiest people among us—marathon runners and their friends and family.

So what about people, like Ann, with cholesterol levels at 200 and above who eat right and exercise? Well, you just can't pick your parents! Heredity is the most important factor in your being able to get your cholesterol level within a good range. To get into that good range, you may need to take one of the statin drugs available that are excellent at controlling your cholesterol, with minimal side effects. There have even been reports that they can eventually dissolve plaque that already exists in your heart that can lead to a heart attack. Given the proven increase in longevity with lower cholesterol levels, it just makes sense to use them. I have found that my patients, active runners, tend to shy away from these drugs because they are sure their running takes care of it. IT DOESN'T! So if after an extensive work-up your doctor prescribes a statin, take it so that you can continue to run far and long for years to come.

In addition to taking a statin, if indicated, for high cholesterol levels, you can stay healthy by putting food onto your Fueling Plates in the proper areas. For example, brightly colored vegetables contain more nutrients to help lower "bad" cholesterol and raise "good" cholesterol. This chapter will also suggest some natural supplements that may help with cholesterol issues.

Cholesterols Defined

Cholesterol is a fat in the blood that is broken down from lipids. You want to prevent high levels of cholesterol and triglycerides, another fat in the blood. Cholesterol and triglycerides are risk factors to clog your arteries. Lowering cholesterol in the blood can help you prevent heart disease and a potential heart attack.

A lipid panel ordered by your doctor does not go by just one number. Total cholesterol is an estimate of all of the cholesterol in your blood, both "good" and "bad" kinds. A total cholesterol number includes each type of cholesterol: triglycerides; LDL cholesterol, a major contributor to clogged arteries; and HDL cholesterol, which actually helps protect against heart disease.

Most guidelines suggest that a desirable level of total cholesterol is under 200 mg/dL. Your total cholesterol level is considered borderline high at 200 to 239 mg/dL and high at 240 mg/dL and up.

Total cholesterol over 240 mg/dL doubles your risk of heart disease. Cardiologists use the 240 mg/dL value as a rule of thumb, and to scare their patients. Regardless of how high your "good" HDL cholesterol is, if your total cholesterol is over 240 mg/dL, you are at risk of heart disease.

I often hear my athletic patients tell me, "My cholesterol is a little high, so I'll just exercise more." Unfortunately, that may not be enough. You could have a "silent" heart problem. If your total cholesterol level is above 200 mg/dL, you should do something about it, starting by making dietary changes or possibly by adding in a cholesterol-lowering medication.

For LDL cholesterol, the optimum level is less than 100 mg/dL. An almost optimal level of LDL cholesterol is 100 to 129 mg/dL, borderline high LDL is 130 to 159 mg/dL, high level of LDL is 160 to 189 mg/dL and very high LDL level is 190 mg/dL and higher. If your LDL cholesterol level is high, your physician will likely recommend lifestyle and dietary changes and a cholesterol-lowering medication. If you are not interested in taking prescription medication at first, carefully watch how much fat you put on your Fueling Plate and increase your exercise levels. To reach your LDL cholesterol goal depends upon other existing risk factors, so you may end up taking prescription medication even if you make lifestyle changes.

Triglycerides are another type of blood fat that is linked to heart disease and diabetes. If your triglyceride level is high, your total cholesterol and LDL cholesterol levels may or may not be high also. If your LDL cholesterol is high, it does not necessarily mean your triglyceride or total cholesterol levels are high. A normal triglyceride level is less than 150 mg/dL, borderline high triglycerides is 150 to 199 mg/dL, and high triglycerides is 200 mg/dL and above.

HDL cholesterol carries LDL cholesterol out of the bloodstream and the arteries. It therefore plays an important role in preventing clogged arteries. Having high levels of HDL cholesterol also has antioxidant and anti-inflammatory effects that help reduce the risk of heart disease. The higher your HDL cholesterol level, the better, even if your total cholesterol level goes up.

An HDL cholesterol level below 40 mg/dL is a risk factor for heart disease for men, and below 50 mg/dL is a heart disease risk factor for women. You have average risk for heart disease if you are a man with an HDL cholesterol level of 40 to 50 mg/dL, and 50 to 59 mg/dL for women. Your HDL cholesterol level is considered high at 60 mg/dL or above for both men and women. As mentioned above, a higher total cholesterol level may be due to high levels of "good" HDL cholesterol, so depending on your other cholesterol levels, discuss with your physician if you need to make any changes to improve your total cholesterol level.

Another type of "bad" cholesterol is very low-density lipoprotein (VLDL) cholesterol. This type of cholesterol has the highest amount of triglycerides. A normal level of VLDL cholesterol is between 5 and 40 mg/dL. The higher your VLDL cholesterol levels, the more likely you are to have a heart attack or stroke. However, a VLDL cholesterol level is not always included in your lipid profile because there is no simple way to measure it. In general, VLDL cholesterol is estimated by dividing your triglyceride level by five. This VLDL cholesterol estimate is not as valid if your triglyceride level is higher than 400 mg/dL.

Be Supplement Savvy

If you are worried about your cholesterol level and have started exercising and eating healthier foods through the Fueling Plates, some natural products may also help improve your cholesterol levels. These supplements can be found in health food stores or the health food section of your pharmacy. However, be aware that these natural products may interact with prescription medications. If you are taking any medication, you must consult with a physician before taking any of these products.

For example, a popular cholesterol-lowering supplement is red yeast rice, which may help lower LDL cholesterol. However, the Food and Drug Administration has warned that red yeast rice products could contain a naturally occurring form of the prescription statin known as lovastatin. Lovastatin in red yeast rice products is potentially dangerous because there is no way to know how much lovastatin might be in a particular product, and there is no way to determine the quality of the lovastatin.

Another potentially dangerous example is niacin. Niacin, also known as vitamin B3, is an important nutrient. In fact, every part of your body needs it to function properly. As a supplement, niacin may help lower cholesterol levels; however, it can also cause serious side effects, such as liver damage, if you take large doses.

Before using any of the following supplements, please discuss them with your doctor. Here's a list of natural ingredients, what they might do to lower cholesterol, and their potential side effects and drug interactions.

- Flax seed may lower LDL cholesterol. It may cause gas, bloating, or diarrhea, and may interact with some blood-thinning medications, such as aspirin, clopidogrel, and warfarin.
- Garlic (one to two cloves of raw garlic per day or 300 milligrams of dried garlic powder in tablet form) may lower total cholesterol and LDL cholesterol. Garlic may lead to a

persistent, distinctive odor on your breath and body, and may interact with certain medications, including blood thinners like warfarin and saquinavir, a drug used to treat HIV infection.

- Green tea or green tea extract may lower LDL cholesterol and triglycerides. It may cause nausea, vomiting, gas, or diarrhea and may interact with blood-thinning medications, such as warfarin.

- Niacin may lower LDL cholesterol and raise HDL cholesterol. The side effects of niacin may include headache, nausea, vomiting, itching, and flushing, which are more common at prescription dose levels.

- Oat bran (found in oatmeal and whole oats) may reduce total cholesterol and LDL cholesterol. Oat bran may cause gas or bloating.

- Omega-3 fish oil (found as liquid oil and in oil-filled capsules) may lower triglycerides. Fish oils may cause a fishy aftertaste, bad breath, gas, nausea, vomiting, or diarrhea, and may interact with some blood-thinning medications, such as warfarin.

- Plant sterols (found in oral supplements and some margarines) may reduce total cholesterol and LDL cholesterol. They may cause nausea, indigestion, gas, diarrhea, or constipation.

- Psyllium, found in seed husk and products such as Metamucil, may lower total cholesterol and LDL cholesterol. It may cause gas, stomach pain, diarrhea, constipation, or nausea, and can reduce absorption of some nutrients, such as iron.

- Soy (found in soy milk, tofu, textured soy protein) may

reduce LDL cholesterol. Soy may cause constipation, diarrhea, bloating, nausea, and allergic reactions.

Fueling Plates for Cholesterol Control

If you are exercising and using the Fueling Plates, with only a small amount of fat on your plate, you are basically doing all you need to help keep your cholesterol levels down.

As you will read in Part 2, the Fueling Plates Program, you can choose foods that are inherently low in cholesterol by putting them in the right section of your Fueling Plate. In general, stay away from fried foods since they contain lots of fat. For example, grilled chicken is better for you than fried chicken. When you put protein onto your Fueling Plate, if it's fried, then some portion of the protein counts toward the fat portion of the Fueling Plate.

We all need some fats in our foods. You want fatty acids, the breakdown products of fats, on board to store energy, just not too much. The idea of the Fueling Plates is not to think so hard about the foods you choose. If you organize the food on your plate as we will describe later, you will have taken cholesterol into account.

If you use the Training Plate, you are eating well to maintain low cholesterol levels. The right foods are incorporated into the Training Plate, so you don't need to worry whether you can eat that food or avoid this other one. Just follow the Training Plate. That's the simplicity of the Fueling Plates program.

Raising HDL Levels

As with all cholesterol levels, HDL cholesterol levels are somewhat determined by your genetics. However, you can naturally increase your HDL cholesterol levels. Here are some ways to raise your HDL cholesterol: consume olive oil; follow a low-carbohydrate diet; exercise regularly; add coconut oil to your diet; stop smoking; lose weight; consume purple-colored fruits and vegetables; eat fatty fish; and avoid artificial trans fats.

Moderate use of alcohol has also been linked with higher levels of HDL cholesterol. For healthy adults, that means up to one drink a day for women of all ages and men older than age sixty-five, and up to two drinks a day for men age sixty-five and younger. However, if you don't drink, don't start drinking to raise your HDL cholesterol levels. Too much alcohol can cause weight gain and might increase your blood pressure and triglyceride levels.

To sum up, cholesterol lowering is important to prevent clogging of your arteries that may result in heart disease. Have your cholesterol levels checked appropriately and follow the Fueling Plates guidelines in Part 2 of this book and exercise regularly. If these lifestyle changes don't work, you may consider taking natural supplements, but don't be afraid of going on cholesterol-lowering medications. Multiple clinical studies show these prescription medications can help you stay healthy, keep your arteries open, and elongate your life.

The next chapter will describe the slew of nutritional supplements now available and help guide you through the aisles of the vitamin store with an easy-to-decipher road map of what works and what to avoid, including the dangers and benefits of various supplements, and little-known and safe performance-enhancing nutrients.

CHAPTER FOUR

Supplements—What Works and What to Avoid

Vitamins and minerals, creatine, caffeine, glucosamine, gingko, amphetamine dangers, diet aids—with all the possible supplements on the market out there, it's no wonder I get so many questions about them! Almost every athlete who comes in to see me asks about supplements. I hear, "My friend is taking this and feels great; should I take it?" or "My friend takes this, can I?" or "What can I take to be better?" They want a magic bullet. The best answer is to eat healthy foods via the Fueling Plates program, exercise regularly, and practice your sport.

For some that's not good enough. They insist on taking a supplement. If you feel you must go to the vitamin store, here are the key supplements often recommended for athletes and my take on them:

Turmeric. Turmeric is a hot new supplement for everyday athletes. It has anti-inflammatory properties, which can help your body recover from a workout faster and may help to prevent injury; may help soothe gastrointestinal distress; and can help optimize liver function and thereby detoxify the body. For runners or those engaged in running sports who suffer from inflamed joints and muscles, consuming turmeric post-workout may help either curb or alleviate the pain.

A spice commonly used in Indian curries, turmeric is a relative to the ginger root family. It is made up of curcumin compounds, which have a powerful anti-inflammatory effect on the body and also have strong antioxidant properties that may help to prevent diabetes, arthritis, Alzheimer's disease, and cancer.

Scientific studies, though not complete, seem to show turmeric can relieve chronic inflammation in osteoarthritic joints. If you have an arthritic joint, try adding ground turmeric to a glass of milk or blend it into a smoothie. The caveat, as always, if you take any medications and add in a supplement, please discuss this with your physician to be sure the supplement doesn't cross-react with any of your medications.

Caffeine. Caffeine increases your body's ability to burn fat while exercising. For those doing endurance events, perhaps the most important benefit of caffeine is that it enhances your body's use of fat as a fuel source, thereby conserving glycogen.

But if you drink too much caffeine before a long bout of exercise, you may make your heart more susceptible to a cardiac arrest. I suggest you limit the amount of caffeine before exercise to the same amount you drink every day, or less than two small cups of coffee, like the size of cup you get at a diner.

I have seen recreational runners down two Red Bulls and several cups of coffee before a marathon in an attempt to lower their time. Are they going to run fast enough to win the race? That's unlikely. Instead, they put themselves at risk of a heart attack to cut off fifteen seconds. It's not worth it.

At a Dallas half-marathon, a forty-four-year-old man who had run many marathons had a sudden cardiac arrest before the finish line. Once we resuscitated him, I found out that he had driven from Chicago to Dallas the day before, drinking high-energy drinks along the way as if they were water. Before the race, he consumed two more of these drinks. At a recent International Marathon Physicians Association meeting, when I interviewed the members about what racers were drinking before a race, I found out each racer who had collapsed and been successfully resuscitated had extra caffeine in his or her system.

Branched chain amino acids (BCAA). BCAAs—leucine, isoleucine, and valine—are essential amino acids but are not produced naturally by the body. These three specific essential amino acids inhibit muscle protein breakdown and aid in glycogen storage.

BCAA supplements are generally associated with bodybuilders, but lately research has shown that runners, especially endurance runners, may benefit from taking BCAA supplements. Some people take BCAA supplements to help them bounce back faster after a workout, reduce muscle soreness, increase power output, increase time to exhaustion, decrease lactate production, and for weight loss.

However, you can likely get enough BCAAs from the food you already eat. You get BCAAs from complete proteins in your diet, such as eggs, meat, poultry, fish, and dairy. Or you can also find them in other plant-based proteins, such as peanuts, chickpeas, lentils, quinoa, and whole grains. When grains and legumes are eaten together (rice and beans or peanut butter on whole-grain bread), they make up a complete protein.

My runners who ask about BCAAs say they have anecdotal evidence that they feel better after a workout when they take supplements. I haven't seen BCAA supplements work one way or the other. Please be aware that supplements aren't regulated, and even though BCAAs don't have any known negative side effects, you always have to be very careful about where you buy them, what's in the supplements, and how much you take. If you decide to take them, carefully follow the directions on the label.

Glutamine supplements. Glutamine is a naturally occurring, non-essential amino acid that is commonly stored in muscles and released into the bloodstream during times of physical stress. Some runners take glutamine supplements to prevent muscle soreness and to improve immune system functioning. Glutamine acts as fuel for immune cells, so when glutamine levels get too low, the immune system may not function optimally.

Most likely you meet the nutritional need for glutamine through your diet. Glutamine is abundant in high-protein foods and select plant sources, including: beef, chicken, pork, fish, eggs, dairy (milk, yogurt, and cheese), cabbage, beets, beans, spinach, peanuts, and barley.

Glutamine supplements can be found in most health food stores in the form of gels or tablets, and glutamine is often an ingredient in many commercial protein powders. There's not much in the sports medicine literature about the benefits of glutamine supplementation if you are otherwise healthy and get adequate nutrition from your diet. Among my patients, I haven't seen it help much.

Probiotics. Probiotics boost the "good" bacteria in your digestive system and help with the absorption of nutrients that fight off "bad" bacteria in the intestines. They may work for a host of digestive issues.

There are different theories for why runners in particular get gastrointestinal upset. During prolonged exercise, blood flow is redirected away from your gut to your muscles to supply oxygen, and to the skin to dissipate heat. This reduced blood supply disrupts the intestinal barrier, allowing toxins to leak into your bloodstream and triggering an immune response. Also, consuming a large amount of carbohydrates to stay fueled during a long exercise bout may lead to malabsorption.

Probiotics may help with both of those problems by maintaining the intestinal barrier and boosting carbohydrate absorption. For example, if you have increased diarrhea, probiotics may help by restoring the balance of bacteria in your gut, and that's a good thing. Some runners take probiotics to prevent going to the bathroom after the first few miles of a race, but they do not work for that. I suggest you talk to a gastroenterologist if you want to take probiotics during exercise.

L-Carnitine. Carnitine is a combination of two essential amino acids, lysine and methionine. The body normally metabolizes carnitine, which is used in the oxidation of amino acids. Carnitine also decreases the levels of lactic acid in muscles during exercise. In athletes, normal carnitine levels drop during intense exercising, and supplements containing carnitine are intended to replace the natural loss of carnitine.

L-carnitine is a naturally occurring amino acid derivative that's often taken as a weight-loss supplement and to boost endurance by runners. It helps to build muscles and breaks down body fats for adenosine triphosphate (ATP) at the same time, and also transports long-chain fatty acids into the mitochondria of cells for energy. The concept is that L-carnitine delivers additional energy by turning your own body fats into ATP, and helps your body create more oxygen-carrying red blood cells.

Some of my patients tell me they use L-carnitine to help with weight loss. I have runners who will run an extra ten miles because they ate a cupcake. Most runners are thin to begin with. I don't believe L-carnitine helps with endurance. The only magic bullet for endurance is training.

Calcium. Calcium plays an important role in strengthening and repairing the bones after a long or hard workout. Since it is the main constituent of bones, it would make logical sense if diminished calcium intake would increase the risk of bone injuries in runners or anyone who plays a running sport, such as triathlon, soccer, basketball, or lacrosse. Calcium also helps your heart muscles pump and transmits signals to your nerves so your muscles contract.

The Institute of Medicine recommends that adults get 1,000 milligrams (mg) of calcium per day. Dairy foods are all rich in calcium, but calcium can also be found in green leafy vegetables (spinach, broccoli, and kale), tofu, almonds, and halibut. You can take calcium supplements, but they may cause negative side effects, for example, calcium carbonate supplements may cause gastrointestinal distress.

A simple blood test will reveal if your calcium levels are low. Some signs of low blood calcium include muscle cramping, brittle nails, numbness in the extremities, irregular heartbeat, and an increase in bone-related injuries. A physician will tell you if you need a calcium supplement for bone health, based on the results of the blood test.

Runners often ask me about calcium supplements because they are worried about their bone health and stress fractures. I tell them the best way to strengthen your bones is through weight-bearing exercise, like running. Taking calcium supplements will not prevent a stress fracture. If you are getting stress fractures, you may have osteopenia (thinning bones) or osteoporosis (bone wasting). Get a bone density test. You may need medical treatment and more than just calcium supplements.

Fish oil. The omega-3 fatty acids found in fish oil protect the cells around your muscle fibers and act as anti-inflammatory agents, which may benefit your muscle function and performance. Studies show taking daily fish oil supplements may reduce muscle soreness, stiffness, and swelling, and improve range of motion. But more research is necessary to confirm these conclusions.

Omega-3 fatty acids are abundant in foods, including fish, seeds, and nuts. Lots of research shows that omega-3 fatty acids can boost your heart and immune system function. I only recommend fish oil for patients with heart conditions who may benefit from a supplement.

Vitamins C and E. The antioxidant vitamins C and E help boost the immune system and fight the oxidative damage that is caused by exercising.

Antioxidant supplementation has become commonplace with endurance athletes. The benefits of an antioxidant-rich diet on enhancing the immune system have been well supported in scientific literature. Numerous supplement companies suggest that antioxidant supplementation may possibly delay fatigue and improve endurance performance; however, the scientific documentation supporting these claims has been lacking.

In fact, recent evidence suggests it may be counterproductive to take antioxidants during endurance activities—the use of vitamin C during physical exercise may actually hinder performance. Without a doubt, more research is needed in this area before I suggest you take vitamin C and E supplements.

Most endurance athletes are already getting sufficient levels of most vitamins, including vitamins C and E. Focus on gaining anti-oxidants through a balanced diet, using the Fueling Plates program.

Magnesium. Magnesium plays a key role in many body processes, including nerve function, blood pressure, immunity, muscle function, bone health, and insulin metabolism. A slight deficiency in magnesium may result in muscle spasms, lactic acid buildup, nerve twitches, cramping, and fatigue.

As with any nutrient, the best source of magnesium is from foods, such as green leafy vegetables (spinach, broccoli, and kale), nuts, seeds (especially pumpkin seeds), peas, beans, lentils, whole unrefined grains, oatmeal, potatoes, halibut, and mackerel. Try to limit consumption of carbonated beverages, sugary treats, caffeine, and alcohol, since they may leach magnesium from your body.

My runners occasionally ask for magnesium supplements to help with muscle contraction in hopes they will run faster. Most people have normal levels of magnesium and do not need supplements. I suggest you get a blood test before taking magnesium supplements. Too high levels of magnesium in the blood can be dangerous. If you take too much magnesium, the symptoms are diarrhea, nausea, vomiting, lethargy, muscle weakness, abnormal electrical conduction in the heart, low blood pressure, urinary retention, respiratory distress, and heart attack. You may need dialysis to flush the excess magnesium out of your kidneys.

Vitamin B12. Vitamin B12, also known as cyanocobalamin, is a man-made vitamin that is important for growth, cell reproduction, blood formation, and protein and tissue synthesis. B vitamins are excreted through urination and therefore are not stored by the body. Vitamin B12 supplements are used to treat vitamin B12 deficiency in those with pernicious anemia and other medical conditions. It can be taken in pill form or injected into a muscle or under the skin.

The vast majority of Americans normally get enough vitamin B12 from meats, fish, and shellfish. If you are eating healthy food from the Fueling Plates, you get enough vitamin B12 in your diet. Vegetarians or vegans may need a vitamin B12 supplement.

Some athletes ask for a large injection (1 gram) of vitamin B12 before competitions to improve performance and endurance. However, scientific research shows supplements of vitamin B12 have no effect on athletic performance unless you have nutritional deficiencies. Also, other drugs may interact with vitamin B12, including prescription and over-the-counter medicines, vitamins, and herbal products. Before taking vitamin B12, tell your doctor about all medicines you use now and any medicine you start or stop using.

My basic message about supplements is you generally do not need them unless you are deficient in a specific nutrient. Why do I tell you about all these supplements? Because you may have questions or heard locker-room talk about them. Most supplements do not produce the benefits you may be looking for. In fact, most of them are a waste of money. I tell my patients if you take something and your body does not really need it, your body just excretes it. So, if you are healthy and take unneeded supplements, they are basically excreted in your now very expensive urine. I believe it's better to concentrate on the food you put on your Fueling Plates, which doesn't take that much effort.

Steroids and Other Supplements

Andy, a seventeen-year-old high school baseball player, was a huge fan of Alex Rodriguez. When I first saw Andy, Rodriguez had just come back from being suspended by Major League Baseball for using performance-enhancing drugs. He and his parents, Carl and Nancy, had come to see me because they knew I took care of both professional and amateur athletes. "I want to take what A-Rod took," said Andy. I spent an hour with Andy and his parents, explaining the danger of taking performance-enhancing drugs and the multiple, lingering side effects of steroids, and told them I would not prescribe them.

"As soon as I heard that my testicles might shrink, I didn't want to use steroids," said Andy. "Dr. Maharam suggested I use the Training Plate and bulk up on the protein portion to help build more muscles, and to add some whey protein to shakes to get in even more protein. I did that over the off-season and put on ten pounds of muscle."

I often give talks to high school, college, and professional athletes with information concerning use, abuse, and potential adverse consequences of steroids, nutritional supplements, and other substances believed to augment or enhance training routines or performance. No talk, however, can serve as a substitute for personalized professional consultation. Consequently, I recommend you do not take any substances reported or claimed to improve training capacity, to increase strength and endurance, or to improve performance without first consulting with your personal physician or a physician knowledgeable in these areas.

First, you need to understand that there are two types of steroids, the anabolic steroids that are used for bulking up, and corticosteroids, such as cortisone, that have anti-inflammatory and healing properties. These are two different substances, but are often confused by many people.

Anabolic steroids have no healing power whatsoever. Their only medical uses are in rare cases of delayed sexual maturation in males, certain neurological diseases where there is muscle wasting, and to suppress estrogen activity in some forms of cancer of the female organs. Even so, they are widely used by athletes to increase size and strength, bodybuilders, and those who want to be bigger to increase their own self-esteem. There is now no question that mega-doses of steroids, combined with a high protein diet and a heavy weight training program, can bring about fifty to sixty pounds of muscle weight gain.

The use of anabolic steroids goes back to the East German and Russian weightlifters and track athletes in the 1960s. Their sudden prominence necessitated the rest of the world's elite athletes to try to catch up. Over the years, anabolic steroid usage spread to athletes in colleges and more recently to high schools and even middle schools, where it has become one of the two greatest substance abuse problems (the other one is alcohol abuse).

The latest surveys show as many as 10 percent of all male high school students will be on steroids at some point over their four years, and at any moment, up to 400,000 students are using steroids. Interestingly, the largest increase in steroid use has been among non-athletes who feel size is important for their self-esteem.

When taken in high dosages, these drugs are extremely dangerous, with a wide range of side effects. Not everyone will get all of the side effects; however, we are not able to predict who will get which effects, when they will occur, and at what point they will be irreversible.

The prototypical anabolic steroid is testosterone, the hormone produced by the testicles in men. Testosterone has two separate, but related, effects. One is the anabolic effect, which is to build muscle size, lean body mass, and body weight, which in turn may provide greater strength and speed. The other effect is the androgenic, or masculinizing, effect, which accounts for normal male characteristics, including the distribution of facial and body hair, deep voice, and reproductive and sexual function.

Pure testosterone has not been useful as medication or for muscle building or performance enhancement because it is rapidly metabolized by the body. In the laboratory, however, testosterone has been altered in significant ways to prolong its effects and to increase its potency. For example, substitution of molecules in certain locations on the testosterone molecule renders the drug effective when administered by injection into muscle; substitution of another molecule in a similar position renders the drug resistant to inactivation by the liver and, therefore, effective as a pill. As the potency of the anabolic effects has increased, so have the side effects of these preparations.

Under federal law, all synthetic derivatives of the male hormone testosterone, called androgenic-anabolic steroids, are considered controlled substances. The Anabolic Steroid Control Act of 1990 classifies these as Schedule III drugs, requiring a doctor's prescription for use.

The regulation of androgenic-anabolic steroids by the federal government predictably led to their sale or distribution in a "black market." Many of these black-market steroids are unsafe because of the lack of testing and safety controls. They may contain impurities, false dosages, and have other particularly dangerous substances and should be avoided at every turn.

There's no doubt that athletes in certain sports could derive greater benefit from steroids than other athletes. For example, weightlifters, who focus on building muscle mass and strength, probably would benefit from the use of high doses of steroids, whereas a fencer might derive less benefit. In baseball, the additional muscle mass associated with steroids presumably might enable batters to hit the ball farther, but the reduction in flexibility from increased muscle mass might make the player swing and miss more often. Also, the increase in muscle mass associated with steroid use is not accompanied by a corresponding increase in tendon, ligament, or joint size or strength, which increases the risk of serious injury. This is a major problem with the use of steroids.

All steroids have harmful side effects, which vary with the particular steroid, dosage, the method and frequency of use, and the length of time over which it is used. Steroid use includes "stacking," in which several compounds are used at the same time for their additive effects (some athletes have used up to eight compounds simultaneously), and "pyramiding," where the drugs are taken in cycles of increasing then decreasing doses, with periods of no drug use. Other drugs are sometimes used to minimize the side effects of the steroids or steroid withdrawal that may occur when they are stopped. Some of the side effects are reversible, but others are not.

The typical side effects of steroids, starting with the mildest and increasing in severity, may include:

- Development of severe acne over the upper trunk. This will usually clear when the drug is discontinued.
- Male pattern baldness. The hair loss is permanent. I find it interesting that the "ego" steroid users will risk this.

- Changes in sexual characteristics, including testicular atrophy—the testicle no longer needs to produce testosterone due to the injection of large amounts of testosterone; sterility—when the testicle ceases to function, sperm production stops, which is usually reversible over a very long period of time; impotence, which is less common; acute prostatic enlargement, which may be so severe it necessitates surgery to relieve the urinary retention; and gynecomastia, a painful enlargement of breast tissue that can only be relieved by surgical removal.
- Calcium depletion. This softens the bones and increases the risk of fractures.
- Increase in muscle and tendon injuries. Increased muscle mass and weight leads to a greater strain on joints, tendons, and ligaments. Chronic steroid use also directly weakens tendon strength and flexibility.
- Liver disease. Early on, the steroid user will show marked changes in liver function tests, which are reversible when the steroid usage stops. Long-term usage can lead to liver degeneration, which can be fatal. Also, the incidence of primary liver cancer is sixteen times higher among steroid users than non-users.
- Cardiovascular changes. Steroid use causes marked increases in total cholesterol levels and also markedly decreases the level of "good" high-density lipoprotein cholesterol. High cholesterol deposits in the heart arteries has led to an increase in heart attacks among steroid users in their twenties; cardiomyopathy due to deterioration of the heart muscle; and a fairly marked increase in high blood

pressure because of the huge mass of new muscles. This increase in blood pressure can be particularly dangerous when combined with the normal rise of blood pressure during weightlifting.

- Personality change. The use of high doses of steroids leads to very aggressive personality change, the so-called "roid rage." Large amounts of male hormone can cause explosive, violent behavior swings. The changes can vary from very subtle to severe psychosis requiring hospitalization. These changes can include irritability, excessive aggression, mania, paranoia, depression (frequently accompanied by suicidal thoughts), anxiety, and panic.

- Psychological and physical dependence. Steroid use can lead to psychological and physical dependence, which makes it hard to curtail their use. Dependent steroid users may experience a variety of withdrawal symptoms when attempting to stop using. A reasonably common problem could be called "reverse anorexia," in which the steroid user becomes fearful of not continuing to get heavier, more muscular, and more masculine. The loss of previous gains between cycles may spur the steroid user to start another cycle. Counseling is needed to help break the dependency, especially since depression may be a factor when steroids are discontinued.

Females who take steroids may develop all of the above side effects, and may also see sexual changes as well. Also, the calcium depletion is even more severe since women have an increased tendency toward osteoporosis. In addition, there are other effects, all of which are irreversible except for loss of menstrual periods. These side effects include growth of facial hair and change from female to male pattern of body hair; deepening of the voice; and sexual changes, including loss of periods, enlargement of the clitoris, and loss of breast tissue.

Recently, I have seen steroid use moving down to middle school students. This may lead to an additional problem of premature closure of the growth centers and the subsequent loss of four to five inches of potential height.

Steroid-like Nutritional Supplements

There are a host of nutritional supplements on the market, including vitamins, minerals, amino acids, plant derivatives, and other natural and synthetic substances. They come in a variety of forms, including powders, tablets, and liquids. All of the supplements claim to improve an athlete's sense of well-being, strength, or performance in one fashion or another.

I like to draw an initial distinction between supplements that claim to increase testosterone levels and those that do not make such claims, but rather rely upon the particular properties of the supplement to allegedly enhance endurance or strength in some other way. Supplements that increase testosterone levels, if they really do that, should be regarded as steroids.

Androstenedione and DHEA

I was the first one to identify that St. Louis Cardinals' slugger Mark McGwire's use of androstenedione was, in effect, a precursor to testosterone, and that McGwire was cheating while helping to fuel Major League Baseball's steroid era. Androstenedione and its chemical cousin dehydroepiandrosterone (DHEA) both effectively become testosterone because of the way testosterone is produced in the body. DHEA is a naturally occurring hormone which, through interaction with other chemicals in the body, converts into androstenedione. Androstenedione, in turn, by a similar process, converts into testosterone.

The theory behind DHEA-based supplements is that they will produce more androstenedione, which eventually will increase the user's testosterone level. Predictably, the theory behind androstenedione-based supplements is that they, too, will increase testosterone levels, and do so more directly than through an increase in DHEA levels. Precisely because DHEA is one step further removed in the testosterone-production chain, the impact of supplements containing it is more speculative. In fact, there has been very little scientific testing of DHEA supplements, but that hasn't stopped them from being available at quite a high price.

More is known about androstenedione, largely as a function of a study jointly sponsored by Major League Baseball and the Major League Baseball Players Association. The baseball study came on the heels of another study that suggested that testosterone levels were not increased by administration of androstenedione. The baseball study, however, utilized dosage levels significantly above those recommended by the manufacturer, and the results showed increases in testosterone levels among users. This finding indicated that androstenedione, from a practical perspective, should be regarded as a steroid.

Androstenedione is not regulated as a steroid because it is considered a nutritional supplement by the federal government. The Dietary Supplement Health and Education Act in 1994 gave nutritional supplement manufacturers greater freedom to market products as long as they do not claim to prevent, diagnose, treat, or cure an illness or disease. This led to the emergence of the innumerable nutritional supplements you see on the shelves of health food stores, all of which are not subject to any stringent chemical analysis. Now that we know that at least some androstenedione-based products do increase testosterone levels, it may be time for the federal government to revisit whether these products should be placed alongside other steroids covered by the Anabolic Steroid Control Act.

As noted earlier, it appears that you can increase testosterone levels only by taking a dose of androstenedione that exceeds the manufacturer's suggested dosage. That leads to a quandary: if you take androstenedione at the recommended level, you're unlikely to receive any significant benefit; on the other hand, if you exceed the recommended level, you may increase muscle mass at the expense of increased risk of adverse side effects. Since androstenedione-based supplements can be purchased over-the-counter, they are readily available to young people seeking to improve their athletic performance. They may take large, frequent doses and put themselves at risk of serious side effects.

Creatine

A majority of sports nutrition supplements, which total more than $2 billion in annual sales in the United States, contain synthetic creatine supplements. The manufacturers of various creatine products have made extravagant claims for their products related to increases in energy, muscle mass, and endurance. In the scientific literature, there are many conflicting reports concerning the effectiveness of creatine.

Creatine comes from three sources: it's synthesized by the body;

it's found in food; and it can be prepared synthetically. Creatine is composed of three amino acids: glycine, arginine, and methionine. These amino acids are mostly found in protein-rich foods, especially fish and meats. Creatine is stored in muscles as creatine phosphate, a precursor of adenosine triphosphate (ATP), which is the immediate source of energy for muscle contraction. Most people consume approximately one to two grams of creatine in their daily diet, and they produce similar amounts in their bodies, which helps maintain normal energy metabolism.

Athletes use creatine in two ways: to enhance bursts of energy needed for short, intense activity, and as a training supplement. Creatine alone does not appear to increase muscle mass, but by allowing you to train more intensely, it may promote faster and more pronounced muscle growth and strength. On the other hand, there may be dangers associated with rapid muscle growth, as with steroids, which would put athletes at higher risk of injury. The potential dangers of creatine require much more study.

Taking large doses of synthetic creatine increases the level of creatine phosphate in muscles and allows sustained, powerful muscular contractions, and may also delay fatigue after a workout. Creatine appears to increase short-term energy for explosive muscle movements, which can be an asset and may improve your performance in short, high-intensity exercises, such as sprinting. However, sports medicine studies show creatine supplements do not enhance sustained athletic performance and maximum oxygen uptake, and do not enhance hand-eye coordination.

Creatine manufacturers recommend starting with a total daily loading dose of ten to twenty grams a day for five days, followed by a total daily maintenance of two to five grams per day. Increasing the dosage will not increase the positive effects. As with other sub-stances, there is a direct correlation between excessive amounts and the risk of side effects.

Also, creatine manufacturers claim that it's safe to use, but there are no carefully controlled studies on either the effectiveness or side effects related to creatine. Overuse of creatine may put excessive strain on the liver and kidneys, and may also cause acute or severe diarrhea. It's essential that you drink adequate amounts of fluids when taking creatine because it is excreted via the kidneys. Not enough fluid can lead to dehydration and muscle cramping.

Unfortunately, there is very little information available about the manufacture and purity standards of creatine, or its interaction with other supplements or medications. No long-term studies of its use are available. I recommend that if you have kidney disease or other health problems you should not take creatine without a physician's supervision.

Creatine is not unhealthy, but I don't generally recommend it. It may help you bulk up, but increasing the water content between muscles fibers makes them easier to tear, and I have seen many people on creatine who end up hurt all the time.

Other Nutritional Supplements

Ephedrine

Ephedrine is a stimulant that is available without a prescription in a variety of nutritional supplements that purport to improve performance and/or decrease appetite. It is extracted from a Chi-nese herb, and may be called ma huang, ephedra, or "herbal ecstasy."

You may see an increase in performance after short-term use of ephedra, particularly if your performance has been compromised by fatigue or lack of sleep. However, increased doses generally do not lead to enhanced performance and may be dangerous. Some of the severe side effects reported related to the drug include high blood pressure, rapid heart rate, seizures, strokes, heart attacks, and death.

Ephedrine is also associated with psychological side effects, such as increased irritability, anxiety, tremors, paranoia and, in rare instances, a complete break with reality. The psychological effects of the drug often severely impair performance. These drugs can be associated with severe dependency or addiction, and for some people, acquiring and using them becomes their overriding concern for living. Commercial preparations containing ephedrine include "Ripped Fuel," "Ultimate Orange," and "Metabolife," which also contain large amounts of caffeine.

Human Growth Hormone

Human growth hormone (HGH) is a hormone produced by the pituitary gland that is responsible for normal growth and development. Typically, HGH is used as a treatment for children whose height is significantly below normal.

Through rumor and anecdotal information, the idea has spread that this drug is a potent anabolic agent that's associated with few side effects. Therefore, athletes use it to help bulk up. HGH has become much sought after and extremely expensive. Young athletes seeking a competitive edge use HGH, while older men may use growth hormone shots as a substitute for working out.

Studies show HGH may increase fat-free mass and total body water, but does not increase muscle size, body strength, or performance, and for those reasons I do not recommend you use HGH.

Originally, HGH was extracted from the pituitary gland of cadavers, and was associated with a number of deaths, probably related to an infectious agent similar to the one that causes "Mad Cow Disease." Synthetic versions of the hormone are now available, and a large amount of counterfeit HGH also exists, for example, vials labeled Lilly Humatrope that actually contain other drugs, such as human chorionic gonadotropin (hCG). HGH is banned by the International Olympic Committee, Major League Baseball, the National Football League, and the World Anti-Doping Agency.

Human Chorionic Gonadotropin

Human Chorionic Gonadotropin (hCG) is a naturally occurring hormone produced by placentas in pregnant women. It's the drug basis for most pregnancy tests, and also is used to treat infertility. In men, hCG stimulates production of testosterone.

Athletes often use hCG during or after high doses of steroids to reduce the possibility of side effects, such as testicular atrophy, or to avoid the crash after stopping steroid use.

hCG can cause side effects similar to steroids, such as male breast growth, acne, mood swings, and high blood pressure. In young athletes, hCG, like steroids, can stunt growth.

Because of the potentially dangerous side effects, I do not recommend the use of hCG.

Erythropoietin

Erythropoietin (EPO) is a naturally occurring molecule that regulates red blood cell production. A synthesized version is used to treat a number of anemias.

EPO purportedly enhances performance and endurance in

certain sports, but there is little data to confirm this. EPO has been implicated in bicycle racing doping scandals because of its capacity to increase the oxygen-carrying capacity of the blood and to deliver more oxygen to muscles. The serious side effects include the potential for fatal stroke and heart attack. Again, because of the side effects issue, I do not recommend taking EPO.

Some athletes, even recreational ones, feel intense pressure to perform. It's no surprise that they look for an edge when they hear that a friend or teammate has found something useful. But given the potential for severe injuries, the many side effects, and the unpredictability of the results that go along with nutritional substances, you must be extremely careful with what you take. As I stated at the beginning of this chapter, you are much better off eating a healthy diet and adopting the Fueling Plates program, along with a good exercise program and adequate sleep, to obtain your optimum weight and build strength and endurance.

PART TWO

The Fueling Plates Program

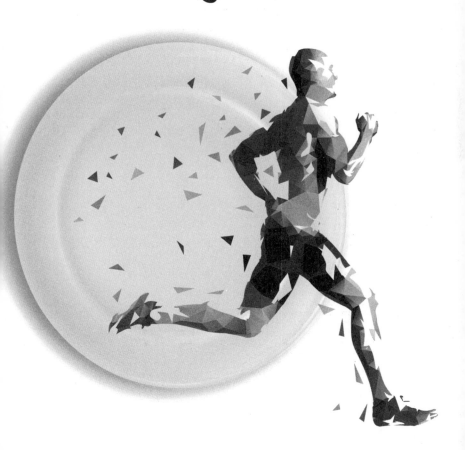

CHAPTER FIVE

How to Use the Fueling Plates Program

Harry, who had run six New York City marathons and a dozen half-marathons, came to see me for a knee problem. I prescribed an orthotic, and as he was leaving the exam room, he asked: "Doc, what should I eat the night before a race?" Back then, in 2012, I suggested he see a sports nutritionist. He came back a month later, and his knee was better, but he said the sports nutritionist was worthless. "She wanted me to change what I eat to nuts and berries," said Harry.

I suggested that Harry separate out the food on his plate into four sections, one for protein, one for fats, one for slow-acting carbohydrates, and the final one for fast-acting carbohydrates. He immediately saw he was eating way too many carbohydrates and not enough protein. Once he adjusted his diet, he had his personal best in the next race. I started using the Fueling Plates concept with all of my patients so they could visually see how to eat right.

*T*his chapter puts down on paper my expertise on how to use sports nutrition concepts to enhance your health. It shows, step by step, how you can apply my revolutionary Fueling Plates program to feel and perform better and have more energy. If you are already exercising, you will get fit faster by eating to fuel your body more efficiently. If you are willing to take advantage of the individualized nutrition program, you will transform your life.

I introduce the four-week Fueling Plates Program to get you eating healthily. The program will sharpen your physiological clues for drinking and eating. Most people have lost the ability to know when they have consumed enough fluid or food. Our bodies have become used to being overstuffed at a meal. You know, when you are full after a holiday dinner: You push back from the table when you can't eat another thing. That's feeling full. I want you to be only 80 percent full. If you're 80 percent full, then you are eating the right amount to maintain weight and fuel your training.

This sounds simple, but it is not dumbed-downed so much that it doesn't work. The greatest reason you don't stick to a diet is that it's too complicated. I got the idea for the Fueling Plates program to be simple from watching commercials for diet plans like Nutrisystem, Jenny Craig, and the South Beach Diet. What do they have in common? They all became successful diet plans because they package the food and send it to you. If you eat their food, you lose the weight. Hopefully, you have a big-enough freezer for a month's worth of food, but you can lose weight. Most diet books are not successful unless they are simple; for example, the South Beach Diet book lists what foods to eat and what not to eat.

I remember my high school biology teacher told me if you understand the minutiae of a biological organism, you will understand the big picture. I understand the minutiae of how to fuel your body for sports, and now I'm giving you the tools for you to learn that, too. But you don't need to learn all the minutiae. Take a leap of faith with me and use the Fueling Plates program. Use it well and you will be eating healthily and performing in the best ways possible.

The key to understanding the Fueling Plates program is that no one size fits all. You are an experiment in and of yourself. This chapter teaches you how to self-experiment using the Fueling Plates to find the right way to eat every day at home, in a restaurant, or at a friend's house. Put food on your plate, then move it into the four appropriate sections. Once you learn and practice this, you will begin to eat healthy and perform your best at the sport you're planning to do.

My patients and those who have heard my talks about sports nutrition all across the world consider me a partner in getting themselves on the path to better eating. Learning how to properly fuel your body through the lens of a sports-medicine professional and taking into account your needs as an active person, you can whip yourself into the best shape of your life.

How to Know When You Are Full

For the Fueling Plates to work, you need to know about fullness. How do you know when you are full yet? When you eat a lot, your stomach stretches. When you feel full, receptors in your stomach send signals to your brain that your stomach has been stretched. However, think about the competitive eater Joey Chestnut, who has won multiple Nathan's Hot Dog Eating Contests. How big is his stomach? He trains by fasting and by stretching his stomach with milk, water, and protein supplements. If Chestnut ate every meal to feel full, he would weigh a ton.

One way to know about fullness is to use the hunger and fullness scale, developed by Linda Omichinski, RD, that describes different levels or varying degrees of hunger and fullness. This tool is designed to help you know when to start or stop eating. Here's the hunger-fullness scale:

Hunger and Fullness Scale	
Hunger	
0–Empty:	Uncomfortably hungry, stomach hurts, headache, difficulty concentrating, fatigue, dizzy, weak, everything sounds good.
1–Ravenous:	Difficulty concentrating, low energy, headache, everything sounds good, past the point of comfortable hunger.
2–Very Hungry:	Stomach growling, stomach may hurt, need to get food now, everything is starting to sound good.
3–Moderately Hungry:	Thoughts about food increase, stomach starts to growl more, need to get something to eat increases.
4–Lightly Hungry:	Starting to think about food, deciding what sounds good to you, what you would like to eat, and maybe stomach gently growling.
5–Neutral:	Neither hungry nor full.

Fullness	
6–Lightly Full:	Satisfied, will likely be hungry again in one to three hours.
7–Moderately Full:	Satisfied, comfortable, will likely be hungry again in two to three hours.
8–Full:	Comfortably full, but would not want to eat more. Satisfied.
9–Stuffed:	Past the point of comfort, full, stomach may hurt.
10–Sick:	Uncomfortably full, feel sick.

If you start eating when you are lightly or moderately hungry, you are more likely to stop eating when you are lightly to moderately full. If you start eating when you are empty or ravenous, you are more likely to eat until you are stuffed or sick. I suggest you eat to number 8, which is about 80 percent full.

This hunger and fullness scale can serve as a guide to help you mindfully connect to your body about when to eat. It can also help you avoid extremes in hunger and fullness, help sustain your energy, and help you feel your best.

Fueling Plates Program

To begin the Fueling Plates program, I want you to get on a bathroom scale in the morning every day. If you see you are gaining weight as you adjust your food intake every day, you're putting too much food on your Fueling Plate and are eating beyond fullness. You need to cut down the height of the food on your Fueling Plate, that is, eat the same healthy foods, but not as much. If you are losing weight, according to your daily weighing schedule, you need to increase the height of the food on your Fueling Plate.

Weigh yourself daily so it becomes a routine. This will be an important practice to follow for the rest of your life. At the beginning of the Fueling Plates program, just knowing you are not gaining or losing weight by the amounts you eat will help you know that the program is working for you. You will accumulate data from your daily weighing and figure out for yourself how much you should be eating. Eventually, you will move food into the four sections on the Fueling Plate with the correct proportions of the proteins, fats, slow-acting carbohydrates, and fast-acting carbohydrates, depending on which Fueling Plate you are using. To begin with, don't try to move food around your plate. Just get the idea of fullness.

You will also practice using thirst as the best mechanism for knowing whether you are dehydrated or drinking too much liquid. Your fluid needs are also individualized and depend on outside factors, such as the heat, humidity, and how far above sea level you live.

Week 1–Drink to Thirst

Can you feel how much your body needs to drink? The old wives' tale you will know when to drink because you're thirsty has been debunked by medical research. Your body needs to be hydrated properly for you to perform your best. This week, I want you to practice using your thirst mechanism to make sure you are hydrated.

A dry feeling in your mouth is your thirst mechanism. For this first week, just think about your thirst. Carry around a water bottle and any time you think you are thirsty, take a sip. Count up how many water bottles you go through each day. Everyone's fluid needs are different, depending on your personal sweat rate, height, weight, and age. Concentrate on thirst to get to know when you are thirsty and feel comfortable in recognizing and then quenching your thirst.

To make sure you are hydrated properly, check the color of your urine, as we discussed in Chapter 2. Your urine should look like lemonade when you are hydrated properly.

Take note of how much you are eating and keep aware of fullness. Observe the height of food on your plate. This will change later based on your goals to decrease or increase weight, or if you are training for or recovering from an event.

Week 2–Eating to Fullness

Jane, a thirty-five-year-old head of marketing at a museum, asked me, "When should I stop eating so I don't eat too much?" I told her about my Fullness Scale, which helps you note how hungry and thirsty you are by answering five simple questions. I explained that midway through a meal, she should ask herself the following questions: Do I feel hungry or full? Am I famished or bloated? Am I thirsty or well hydrated? Does my stomach feel empty or filled to capacity? And, am I comfortable, ready to eat more, or am I uncomfortable and want to push away from the table? Then using a scale of 1 to 5 for each question, Jane should add up her score and divide by five. If it averaged 4, then she was probably full and should stop eating.

"I tried the Fullness Scale at dinner that night and scored a 5. I knew I had eaten too much. I practiced some more the next few days and began to figure out when I was just about full. I soon got the hang of it," said Jane.

How do you know when to stop eating? You need to walk away from the dinner table when 80 percent of your hunger has been satisfied. In addition to the hunger-fullness scale below, I have another very easy way to know if you are full. Near the end of a meal, put your hand on your belly to get a sense of how full you are. If you feel full, like the time when you ate that big steak at a fancy restaurant, then you have eaten too much.

I have also adapted a psychological mood scale to use as a fullness scale. Use the following fullness scale with word pairings, such as "Hungry" versus "Full," to help you know when the feeling of fullness starts, with 1 being the most hungry, thirsty, and so on, to 5 being the most full, hydrated.

Hunger and Fullness Scale				
Hungry				Full
❏ 1	❏ 2	❏ 3	❏ 4	❏ 5
Famished				Bloated
❏ 1	❏ 2	❏ 3	❏ 4	❏ 5
Thirsty				Well-hydrated
❏ 1	❏ 2	❏ 3	❏ 4	❏ 5
Empty				Filled to capacity
❏ 1	❏ 2	❏ 3	❏ 4	❏ 5
Comfortable, Ready to Eat More			Uncomfortable, Want to Push Away from the Table	
❏ 1	❏ 2	❏ 3	❏ 4	❏ 5

This scale can add to your understanding of eating to fullness. How do you know if you are full? Go through each of the word pairings to see how full you feel. Note the number for each of the five word pairings so you don't focus on one set of words, add them up, then divide by five. The larger the number, the fuller you are. Your goal is to reach an average of 4 on the fullness scale. When you reach 4, you will have satisfied 80 percent of your hunger.

You can also use the information on your weight that you have gathered to better understand the word pairings. You will know if you're 2 out of 5 on the scale, it's likely you are not eating enough. If you are at 5, you're likely eating too much.

With this better understanding of fullness, now experiment as to how high to pile the food on your plate. Visualize how much food to put on the Fueling Plates to achieve fullness. If you are 3 on the fullness scale, you are somewhat hungry. If you are 4 on the scale, you are not hungry; you are full. If you are 5, it's time to stop eating. I would like you to not get to 5. Aim for 4 on the fullness scale.

Week 3–Drawing the Plates

Your only job this week is to practice drawing the four different Fueling Plates—the Healthy Plate, Training Plate, Night-Before-an-Event Plate, and After-a-Long-Workout Plate. Start by keeping a diagram of the Healthy Plate with you at dinner. Take your fork and move the food around to match the diagram. Any excess food should be separated out and put aside as leftovers. Within one week of practice, you will be able to draw the plate without the diagram. Then you can practice how high to build each section of the plate for fullness.

Let's imagine the Healthy Plate for a meal of chicken and pasta with piccata sauce plus green beans with mandarin orange slices. The chicken is your protein, the pasta is your slow-acting carbohydrate, the mandarin orange is your fast-acting carbohydrate, and

Healthy Plate

Training Plate

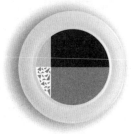

Night-Before-an-Event Plate

After-a-Long-Workout Plate

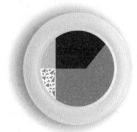
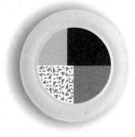

Legend: light gray = low fat; black = protein; dark gray = slow-acting carbs;
speckled = fast-acting carbs

the piccata sauce is your fat. If the amount of chicken you cooked goes over the lines allotted for protein, cut down on the amount of chicken. If the spaghetti creeps over to other parts of plate, cut back on it. If you were to eat this meal in a restaurant, I would suggest you ask for the sauce on the side because the piccata sauce is mostly fat. It's a lot harder to tell how much fat is in a dish if the sauce is already on it. It's easier for you to see how much to put in the fat section of your Healthy Plate if you have the sauce on the side. The mandarin orange slices fill out the fast-acting carbohydrate portion of the Healthy Plate.

Week 4–Which Plate to Use

This week, you will practice which plates to use and when to use them. You will use a different Fueling Plate for different times of your training. The Healthy Plate is your everyday eating plan. The Training Plate helps you gain strength and endurance as you train. The Night-Before-an-Event Plate adjusts eating to meet upcoming demands. For example, if you are doing a long run, you need to eat more slow-acting carbohydrates. If you have an early-morning tennis match, you need more fast-acting carbohydrates. The After-a-Long-Workout Plate adjustments help you recover quickly.

If you are not exercising and have not set any goals, the first thing is to start exercising. If you exercise on the weekend to maintain a healthy lifestyle, not to compete, and just want to maintain your current weight, use the Healthy Plate. If you want to lower or raise your weight, use the Healthy Plate. You want to maintain a low-fat diet, so just decrease or increase vertically the amount of food on your plate.

Say you are exercising and training for an event. The Training Plate has a little more of the slow-acting carbohydrates and less fast-acting carbohydrates to build up stored energy in glycogen than the Healthy Plate. You will still need fast-acting carbohydrates during exercise, but you need more slow-acting carbohydrates on board so that you have stored energy. The Training Plate has about the same amounts of protein and fat as the Healthy Plate.

Notice that the Night-Before-an-Event Plate has less protein and more stored energy than the Healthy Plate. I want you to have enough glycogen on board so your body doesn't have to use up stored protein. When you hit the wall during a long event, you will have used up all the carbohydrate stores, and your body will start to use protein and fats for energy. It's better to use carbohydrates because they provide the most efficient use of energy in a long bout of exercise in an endurance-type event.

The Night-Before-an-Event Plate is very important. For example, runners were known to carbo load the night before a long-distance race. They would eat huge amounts of pasta and leave out much-needed protein, which is broken down to available amino acids to build back muscles during exercise. When you don't eat protein, you don't have the amino acids available to do this important reconstruction afterwards.

On the other hand, if you eat too much protein, you may feel tired during the event. That's what often happens on Thanksgiving when you eat lots of turkey and feel so full and tired. It's why you do not want to eat so much protein the night before a long event.

The After-a-Long-Workout Plate is designed for use when you have used up your carbohydrate stores and you are tired. At this point, you need a little more protein and little more fat to build back your energy. The additional fast-acting carbohydrates will counteract your feeling of exhaustion. Also, you need more slow-acting carbohydrates to replenish your glycogen stores. The slight excess of fast-acting carbohydrates will also be converted to glycogen.

While you may eat more protein in the Training Plate and the Night-Before-an-Event Plate, you don't need that much protein for the After-a-Long-Workout Plate because most people tend to get nauseous when they eat so much protein after a long event.

When you start using the Fueling Plates at first, have the diagrams of the four plates with you when you eat to make sure you are eating the right foods. This works to help you know you are eating healthily, and helps reinforce what is a slow-acting carbohydrate, a fast-acting carbohydrate, protein, or fat.

It only takes four weeks to ingrain the concept of the Fueling Plates. By then, you will have all the skills you need to use this concept for the rest of your life. It will become a habit, and you will now have the skills to use it. You won't even have to think about it. Just move the food to the proper section on the plate you are using. You can feel confident about what you are eating to keep you healthy and not throw off your training before or after an event.

If you are out with an injury, go back to the Healthy Plate. Once you're back in training, use the Training Plate, and other plates as necessary. The Fueling Plates program makes you an efficient eater of the fuels you need to perform your best.

Next, we go into the health benefits of the Healthy Plate.

CHAPTER SIX

The Healthy Plate

Richie, a thirty-year-old lawyer and one of my running patients, wanted to know how to eat better, so I showed him how to use the Healthy Plate. "That is not going to work for me. I use an online service to deliver all my food right to my door. I don't shop in markets," Richie told me. I laughed and said, "You can have all your foods brought in by a diet company, but if you really want to be healthier, you will have to shop for yourself."

Richie agreed to make time to go to the local market and buy his own food for one week. "I did not know how great the market is. There are beautiful fruits and vegetables and more stuff than they have online. This is the most fun I have had in months, and I feel great, too. I can't wait to go back and shop again," said Richie.

This chapter highlights the **Healthy Plate.** I show you how to maintain a healthy weight and get all the nutrition you need from all the proper food categories. The Healthy Plate keeps things simple—eat a little more than half of your calories from protein at every meal, only 10 percent from fast-acting carbohydrates, which are used up immediately; 30 percent from slow-acting carbohydrates, which are stored in the form of glycogen; and a small amount from heart-healthy low fats, just enough for energy but not too much to clog the arteries.

These percentages are derived from sports science research that says the healthiest diets contain about 50 percent protein for muscle building, 10 percent fast-acting carbohydrates for fast energy, 30 percent slow-acting carbohydrates for endurance, and that are low in fats for additional energy. You don't need to be absolutely precise in these percentages, just approximate as best you can.

Take a look at the diagram of the Healthy Plate. As you examine it, take the empty plate in front of you and draw a mental picture of the Healthy Plate on it. Put a tablespoon or so of food into each of the four sections on the plate—protein, slow-acting carbohydrates, fast-acting carbohydrates, and fat. Then continue to fill up various sections of the plate.

HEALTHY PLATE

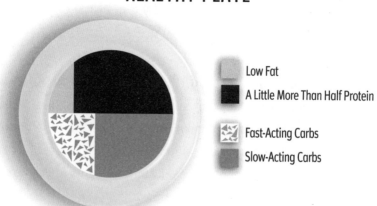

Low Fat

A Little More Than Half Protein

Fast-Acting Carbs

Slow-Acting Carbs

Just visualize the Healthy Plate and put your food in the designated sections; you don't have to calculate exactly. That's one of the advantages of the Fueling Plates program. You don't need to get out your cell phone and calculate how many calories are on your plate, or a scale to weigh the food, as you must in some diet programs.

We are not talking about keeping track of calories or grams of weight. Each exerciser is an individual and has individual nutritional needs. A gymnast might fill up the four sections of the Healthy Plate very thinly, while a defensive tackle in football would pile the food up high. You need to know your goal—to lose weight, maintain weight, or gain weight—to know how much food to include.

The makeup of your Healthy Plate, as well as how much food should be heaped on the plate, can be readily determined. There is no one-size-fits-all approach because the environment, your metabolic rate, and activity level can all dictate your nutritional needs. One thing is for certain: what you put into your mouth—and when and how much—can make or break your workout experience.

Vegetarian Healthy Plate

Jennifer, a thirty-five-year-old banker, decided to stop eating meat and become a strict vegetarian. "I am eating tons of salad and feel great except in regard to my running. Now when I run long distances, I am getting tired quicker and my times are increasing. My usual aches and pains after a long run now last two days. I used to recover quickly, usually within one day," said Jennifer.

I suggested that Jennifer use the Healthy Plate, with some modifications. "In order to be my healthiest, I needed to know the top food choices for vegetarians. Once I knew those, it was easy to incorporate them into the Healthy Plate. Now my energy level is back, and I'm running faster than ever," said Jennifer.

A vegetarian diet has been proven to have health benefits, such as reducing your risk of heart disease, diabetes, and some cancers, including cancers of the stomach, colon, and lungs. The best definition of a vegetarian diet is a diet free of meat, fish, and fowl. Lacto-ovo vegetarians do not eat animal flesh but eat eggs and milk products. Vegans do not eat any animal-based products, including honey. Pescatarians eat fish and seafood.

The number one cause of tiredness in new vegetarians is their lack of focus on eating enough carbohydrates, protein, iron, calcium, zinc, vitamin B12, riboflavin, alpha-linolenic acid, and vitamin D. Here are some ways to incorporate these nutrients into your diet. Emphasize them when you are filling up your Healthy Plate if you are a vegetarian.

Carbohydrates. This is your body's fuel. If you don't have enough carbohydrates, your energy level as well as your endurance will decrease. Vegetarians can consume carbohydrates by eating whole grains found in barley, whole-wheat pasta, whole-grain breads, and brown rice. Other excellent sources of carbohydrates are whole fruits, squash, beans, corn, sweet potatoes, lentils, and quinoa. If you eat dairy, then milk, cheese, and yogurt are good sources of carbohydrates.

Protein. Proteins break down to amino acids, which are the building blocks for all structures within the body. If you don't have enough protein, it takes longer to repair microtears that occur during exercise. That's why Jennifer's post-event muscle soreness probably lasted two days instead of one. Try to eat more high-protein grains such as quinoa, beans, nuts, and nut butters. Veggie burgers that are labeled with 5 grams of protein or more are an excellent choice, as well as eggs, if you eat them. Tofu and edamame are the favorite choice of protein for some of my vegetarian patients.

Iron. Iron is an important part of the red blood cell as it carries oxygen from your lungs to the rest of your body. Low iron results in anemia and tiredness. The best iron-rich choices include dried apricots and prunes, soy-based foods, fortified breakfast cereals, whole-wheat breads, beans, nuts, and eggs, if you eat them.

Calcium. Calcium is important for good bone health. You can get this nutrient in tofu, sesame tahini, almonds, calcium-fortified almond or soy milk, and green leafy vegetables, like spinach and kale. If you eat dairy, you can find calcium in milk, yogurt, and cheese.

Zinc. Zinc is an important booster of the immune system. New vegetarians often complain they seem to get sick more than they used to. Try adding soy milk, soybeans, nuts, seeds, mushrooms, split peas, lentils, and black-eyed peas to your Healthy Plate.

Vitamin B12. Vitamin B12 deficiency can lead to anemia and cause tiredness. Vegetarians should try to eat some fortified breakfast cereals and soy-based beverages to keep vitamin B12 at an adequate level. Since vitamin B12 is found naturally only in animal products, if you can't eat the above, buy a B12 supplement at a health food store and take it daily to increase your energy level.

Riboflavin (Vitamin B2). Riboflavin is a vitamin that helps the body break down carbohydrates, protein, and fats to produce energy. It fundamentally allows oxygen to be used by the body. If you don't have enough riboflavin, again, you can feel tired. Riboflavin is found in soy milk, mushrooms, almonds, and fortified breakfast cereals. If you eat dairy, cow's milk and yogurt are rich in riboflavin. If you can't eat enough of these foods, try getting a vitamin B2 supplement at a health food store.

Alpha-linolenic acid (Omega-3). Omega-3 is a fatty acid that helps boost the immune system. Research has shown that omega-3 fatty acids enhance B cells (a type of white blood cell). Lack of it may contribute to you getting sick more often. Omega-3 fatty acids can be found in tofu, soybeans, walnuts, canola, and flaxseed oil.

Vitamin D. Vitamin D is important for bone health as well as immune, muscle, and nerve function. It is known as the sunshine vitamin because our bodies make and absorb vitamin D from exposure to the sun. If you can't get outside, try eating mushrooms, fortified breakfast cereal, fortified orange juice, and soy and almond milk.

Maximize Color

How do you know if the foods you eat are healthy or not? My friend Thomas Keller, the chef/owner of Per Se restaurant in New York City, says the best way to know is by color. If the color of the food is bright, it's more likely to be healthy for you. This is the best advice I have ever heard from any type of medical professional, sport nutritionist, or chef.

Simple, bright food keeps everything healthy, as long as it is not overcooked, which may destroy the nutrients. You need to learn to trust yourself to pick out fresh produce. Here's a little game to help you learn to trust yourself. Go to the market's produce aisle with two plastic bags. Pick out some apples, carrots, string beans, and green peppers. In one bag, put the brightest, most colorful produce and in the other bag put in the dullest ones you can find. Buy both bags, take them home, and put the bright food on one plate and the dull food on another plate. You can see it makes a difference when you pick colorful fruits and vegetables. Now you will be more than comfortable enough to put healthy food on your plate and maximize your color.

Feeling of Fullness

For the Healthy Plate, I want you to practice the feeling of fullness for dinner. There are four ways in which your body and brain understand when you are full. This feeling of fullness is called *satiety*. One is the expansion of your stomach, which we discussed in the previous chapter. The second is a sensory experience—the appearance, smell, taste, and texture of the food you are consuming will help you know whether you are full or not. The third way involves mental beliefs about how filling the food is. If you eat a salad and think it is "diet food," you may not feel as full as if you ate a big bowl of macaroni and cheese. Yes, macaroni and cheese is heavier and will fill up your gut, but the psychological component adds to your knowledge that you will be full. The fourth and final way is through hormones released during absorption and digestion of food. There are hormones that tell the brain how much fat is stored in the body, which affects your fullness over the long-term. These signals come together in areas in the brain controlling energy and food intake.

Although you feel your stomach filling up as you eat, it can take some time for these fullness signals to reach the brain. Everybody is different in how much time it takes to get these signals of fullness to the brain. Despite sophisticated hormonal mechanisms about the feeling of fullness, some people still eat when they feel full or resist eating when they are hungry.

Eating Behavior Influences

Seven factors influence eating behavior as well as the body's signals of fullness. These include:

1. Palatability of food—how much you like the taste of the food you are eating. If the food tastes really good, you may end up getting to the point where you feel like, "I'm stuffed. I can't eat any more." The goal is to stop before you get to this point.

2. Portion sizes. Some people like to fill up their plate, while others limit the amount of food they eat. This is individualized. How high you pile the food on your Healthy Plate is determined by your goals: whether to maintain, lose, or gain weight.

3. Variety of food and drinks. Psychological cues influence what you eat. If you eat a food you have never had before, you tend to want to have more of it.

4. Your emotional state. Comfort foods are childhood meals you have an emotional attachment to. Maybe they remind you of your grandmother, who made the world's best meatloaf and mashed potatoes with gravy on Sunday afternoons. You can't wait to have them when you are feeling

blue—and want to keep eating them. Be aware of the emotional attachment to that food, or going to a specific, favorite restaurant.

5. Aspects in your surroundings. Advertisements make you want to eat more. If you see a television commercial, complete with mouthwatering pictures about a new fast-food sandwich, you may not only go there to eat the sandwich but unwittingly eat way past when you are full because the aroma of fries and the value of the full meal deal are too good to pass up.

6. Social situation. When you eat with family or friends, either at home or in a restaurant, often you do not think about how much you are eating. Or, the portion size is so big, and you don't want to leave food on your plate. Fill up the Healthy Plate and understand that you can save any extra food or take it home with you.

7. Physical activity level. If you run twenty-five miles a week, you will need to eat more than if you run five miles a week. Exercise increases your metabolic rate as compared to someone who is a sofa spud. Top athletes often eat multiple meals a day to replace the calories they use during exercise.

Being Healthy

Walter, a sixty-four-year-old school teacher, played tennis one night a week in a long-time doubles game and had a regular singles game on weekends, too. "I started using the Healthy Plate to keep up my energy levels. We always go out to eat after we play. My buddies complained at the restaurant that I was playing with my food like a three-year-old," said Walter. "I told them, 'The end justifies the means. I feel good about the food I eat, and I feel healthy, so get over it.' I tell the waiter, 'I'm on a special diet and can only eat this much. The rest is going home with me.'"

Being healthy means not only are you physically healthy but mentally and socially healthy as well. The World Health Organization (WHO) definition of health is "a state of complete physical, mental, and social well-being and not merely the absence of disease or infirmity." I totally agree with this definition. It's always good to have something in writing to back up any discussions on the Healthy Plate.

Here's how the Healthy Plate backs up the WHO definition of health:

- **Physical**—The Healthy Plate provides the proper nutrients in a balanced manner to give you the health benefits of eating properly.
- **Mental**—You know that you are on the right course if you use the Healthy Plate. If you are eating well with the Healthy Plate, you won't feel tired after a huge meal. You know it's working for you because you have more mental energy and you feel sharper in everyday life.
- **Social well-being**—Using the Healthy Plate puts you in a better frame of mind. If you use the program, you won't feel hungry and be grumpy. You will be better at interacting with others. If you feel good about the foods you eat, you will be more personable with friends and family in addition to feeling good about yourself.

In the next chapter, we will go into detail about what to eat during training by using the Training Plate.

CHAPTER SEVEN

The Training Plate

Leah was training to run a 5K charity event and was thinking about ordering Nutrisystem or Jenny Craig to lose some weight. "I know these diets are not good for me as an athlete, but I don't have time to understand everything in nutrition books," said the forty-year-old accountant, who plays tennis on weekends and takes Zumba and Spinning classes at her health club during the week.

I asked Leah if she knew what a fat is, and she said correctly, "It's something oily." I told her she wanted a low-fat diet and if she sees oil or butter on food to push that food to the top left corner of her plate. Next I asked her about protein. "Meat," she said. Perfect. Vegetarians can think about tofu, too. I explained why protein is important for an athlete—to rebuild ligaments and soft tissue microtears that occur when she works out.

"The most important thing is your fuel, which is your carbohydrates," I said. Simple sugars that taste sweet are called fast-acting carbohydrates. The more sugary it tastes, the more useful it is right away. Slow-acting carbohydrates are not as sweet and provide fuel for later use.

Then I drew the Training Plate. "Fit your food into these four areas. That's all you have to do," I told Leah. "You don't have to weigh your food *or count calories or learn the glycemic index numbers. Just make most of your plate protein and slow-acting carbohydrates."*

T raining is really practice for an event, and the event is really a celebration of your training. To train your body properly for an event, you need to eat from the Training Plate.

It's important to know what you're eating, particularly if you're working out regularly or training for a specific event. I have synthesized the glycemic index numbers into something that is simple to follow. Remember, as noted in the Introduction, the glycemic index gives you a way to tell slower-acting carbohydrates from faster-acting carbohydrates. The breakdown of the three most important foods on the Training Plate comes from nutrition literature about what everyone agrees on what an athlete should be eating while training.

This chapter will also cover the instant energy gels, those tempting yet artificial, candy-looking packages of concentrated sugar that can be deployed for success or can have you running not only a literal marathon but a "metabolic marathon" as well.

The Training Plate

The Training Plate should consist of about half of the calories from protein, slightly less than half from slow-acting carbohydrates, and only very small percentages of fast-acting carbohydrates and fat.

Compared to the Healthy Plate, while training, most people need more protein than they normally would eat because, during

TRAINING PLATE

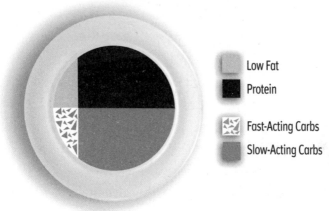

- Low Fat
- Protein
- Fast-Acting Carbs
- Slow-Acting Carbs

aerobic activity for a sustained time, they quickly use up the sugar in fast-acting carbohydrates. You need glycogen to turn into sugar to maintain aerobic activity. Unlike the Healthy Plate, you need to make sure to concentrate more on protein because you are breaking down protein every day you train.

You also need to add in some fast-acting carbohydrates to build up glycogen needed for training, and cut down slightly on slow-acting carbohydrates while maintaining similar levels of protein and fat as the Healthy Plate.

Training to Be Full

To get the most out of the Training Plate, you need to figure out how much to eat to fullness, not bursting and not feeling hungry, when you get up from the table. In time, it's easy to know what your body needs. You have already practiced this with the Healthy Plate.

So how high should you pile up each section of the Training Plate? That depends on how full you are and the amount of training you are doing. As I described earlier (see Chapter 2), the first step is to know when you are thirsty and to use the dry feeling in your mouth as a thirst mechanism. Once you are comfortable with the concept of recognizing your thirst, then you will move on to feeling comfortable when you are eating food.

By now, you should feel good about recognizing the fullness in your stomach, placing your hand on your belly where the ribs end on the right side of your torso. If you feel a strong push-back on your hand, you have eaten enough. If you feel a weak push-back, you can eat more. You will be surprised at how soon you will know when you are full and have eaten enough at dinner. If you feel full, it's time to stop eating. If you're out at a restaurant, bring the food home with you. If you're home, put it away as leftovers for another time.

With the Training Plate, now you can practice that full feeling at breakfast and lunch as well as dinner. This feeling may be more subtle since you likely don't eat as big a breakfast or lunch as dinner, and you may not feel as full. Practice this, and you will start to understand when you're full or not, and then apply it to all meals. You can continue to do this for the rest of your life.

If you train more than once a day or more than a few hours total, then you may need to pile more food on each section of the Training Plate. If you burn more calories in training, you need to replenish those nutrient supplies you have depleted. Don't go overboard. Just add a little bit more, in particular, protein and slow-acting carbo-hydrates, to make sure your body continues to get the nutrients it needs to train hard.

Training Plate Food

A good training diet contains, for example, some pasta or baked potato with a low-fat sauce like pomodoro, or broiled, skinless chicken with a low-fat sauce like vinaigrette, fresh vegetables, and a refined grain such as bread or brown rice. You also need some fresh fruit for slow-acting carbohydrates, such as oranges, grapes, strawberries, raspberries, or melon.

The Training Plate already accounts for food you will find in the glycemic index. The glycemic index is on a sliding scale along a continuum. On the left are the lowest glycemic foods, such as beans, and on the right are the highest glycemic foods, such as chocolate. Pasta with beets is in the middle. The beauty of the Fueling Plates program is you don't need to know the actual glycemic index number. All you need to know is if a food is a slow-acting carbohydrate or a fast-acting carbohydrate.

Slow-acting Carbohydrates

100 percent stone-ground whole-wheat or pumpernickel
Oatmeal (rolled or steel-cut), oat bran, muesli
Pasta, converted rice, barley, bulgur
Sweet potato, corn, yam, lima/butter beans
Peas, legumes, and lentils
Most fruits, non-starchy vegetables, and carrots

Medium-acting Carbohydrates

Whole-wheat, rye, and pita bread
Quick oats
Brown, wild, or basmati rice, couscous

Fast-acting Carbohydrates

White bread or bagel

Corn flakes, puffed rice

Bran flakes, instant oatmeal

Short-grain white rice, rice pasta

Macaroni and cheese from mix

Russet potato, pumpkin

Pretzels, rice cakes, popcorn,

Saltine crackers

Melons and pineapple

Sweets and sweetened fruit (for example, glazed apples)

If you eat slow-acting carbohydrates, it takes longer for your body to break down the food into simple sugar for cells to use as energy. If you eat fast-acting carbohydrates, the break-down process is shorter in both time and the amount of reactions that have to happen to reduce the food to simple sugar.

Why a Training Plate?

Why do you need the Training Plate while training? The answer is so that you can train at your best and get the best result in your upcoming event. No matter what sport you play, you will refurbish your protein stores quicker with the Training Plate and get the proper nutrients to perform at your peak. Also, if you eat properly, you will feel less post-event muscle soreness and for a shorter time because your muscles are repairing at a rapid rate.

What's more, when you eat from the Training Plate, you not only fuel the movements necessary for your sport, but also ensure that other body parts get the proper nutrients, too. When you play a running sport for a long period, your blood flow is redirected into the legs. If you don't eat enough protein during the day, then there will be no nutrients available to your kidneys, brain, upper extremities, mucous membranes, and body fluids.

What to Eat Before an Event

You can also use the Training Plate to choose high-powered foods before an event. Two hours beforehand, you want a combination of slow-acting carbohydrates, fast-acting carbohydrates, protein, and even some fat. My favorite pre-event meal is what I call the "Elvis bagel," based on Elvis Presley's favorite breakfast. Eat a bagel (slow-acting carbohydrates), a banana (plain, not fried like Elvis, which contains fast-acting carbohydrates), and peanut butter (some protein and a little fat).

I recommend you eat a salt bagel if you have trouble knowing how much water to drink during the event. The extra salt will help prevent muscle cramping during a long event by keeping the salt level in your blood high enough to allow your muscles to work efficiently.

Other pre-event options include an egg on a bagel with some fruit jam, along with some orange slices or a handful of berries. Mix and match foods, so long as you fill up the Training Plate diagram with the proper amount of slow-acting carbohydrates, fast-acting carbohydrates, protein, and fat.

Instant Energy Gels

I see lots of running events that hand out instant energy gels, what I call "goo," to everyone. These small, gooey packets contain very high amounts of sugar for so-called instant energy. But if you use them too much, too often, you run the risk of running a "metabolic marathon." Here's what I mean by metabolic marathon. Every time you take a high amount of sugary substance into your stomach, your body responds by releasing insulin to send the sugar into the body's cells to be used as energy. Once your body metabolizes the sugar, you become hungry for more high-sugar food. If you keep downing "goo," your blood sugar levels keep bouncing up and down with the release of insulin, your cells work harder, and it's as if your body is running a metabolic marathon. The overall effect of too much "goo" is you feel worse afterward.

If you insist on using "goo," use it just once after the middle of the event to give you a final push toward the finish, for example, around the fifteen-mile mark of a marathon, after two sets of tennis, or at halftime of a soccer or basketball game. Take only one packet of the prearranged dose.

I would prefer to see you use oranges. If you went to a buffet and had a choice of cut-up oranges or "goo," which would you put on your plate? I hope your answer is oranges. They are a natural, fast-acting carbohydrate food. Soccer players often need an extra boost of sugar. That's why savvy soccer moms and dads know to hand out orange slices to young players during breaks in the action.

What to Drink and Eat on Game Day

What should you drink on game day? Drink to thirst, as you have practiced. If you are running a marathon, don't stop and drink at every water stop. If it's a hot day, you're better off pouring some of the water over your head. Research shows if you drink at every water stop, you can develop hyponatremia. Hyponatremia occurs when the level of sodium in your blood is abnormally low. Drinking too much water during endurance sports may cause the sodium in your body to become diluted. This is a dangerous condition that can cause your brain to swell and even lead to death.

You don't need to eat much during an event. Most athletic events are three to four hours, tops. Eating from the Training Plate will provide you with enough carbohydrates to get you through a long event. I have seen walkers who take ten hours to complete a marathon, eating a bag of Doritos or potato chips as they cross the finish line. That's because they're hungry and need food! They would be better off with homemade gorp, a combination of fast-acting carbohydrates like raisins or dried fruit, added salt from nuts to prevent cramping, and chocolate nibs for a little burst of energy.

With the Training Plate, if you follow the breakdown of foods, you will have balanced your body's nutrition for your sport. Your body will remain healthy, and the parts of the body that need to be at their strongest will have the nutrients they need to perform. Eating will not be an issue in your performance. Lack of technique or natural ability, improper training, and not having proper nutrients and fuel on board can all lead to a poor performance during an event. But eating from the Training Plate eliminates the potential nutrition problem since you will be properly fueled.

The Training Plate is great for training right up to the night before a long event. The night before, you need to increase your carbohydrates to prepare for the event in the Night-Before-an-Event Plate, which I discuss in the next chapter.

CHAPTER EIGHT

The Night-Before-an-Event Plate

I was at the start of the New York City Marathon in 2017, and then got a lift to the end of the race. After finishing the race, many runners need to go to the bathroom. There was a huge line of runners at the portable toilet at the finish line. I asked the runners in line for the toilet what they had eaten the night before the race, and they all said, "I ate pasta; I ate great." Only a few had eaten some protein. Most had spaghetti and red sauce with no protein and ate more than they normally would to "carbo load." If they had eaten the amount of food as they usually did and added in some protein, chances are they wouldn't have been waiting in that long line.

The night before a big event is not the time to throw a pasta party. This chapter debunks the "carbo loading" myth. To prevent post-event muscle soreness and repair your muscles the next day, you need some protein the night before, not just pasta.

The Night-Before-an-Event Plate raises slow-acting carbohydrates to more than half of the total calories, but keeps fast-acting carbohydrates and fat at the same levels as the Training Plate, while cutting back slightly on protein. Too much fat, for example, a big dinner of spaghetti and meatballs, before an event and you're likely to need a bathroom break during the next day's long event.

I spend a lot of time at the start line at races. At the New York City Marathon, at the first bathroom, there's always a long line. I ask people what they ate the night before, and 99 percent say they only ate pasta, no protein. Their reason for stopping is not bad training, but bad meal planning. With the right proportions, you will feel healthy the night before and the next day because you planned to eat so you were fueled correctly.

What's so important about eating the night before, and why do I slightly adjust the proportions for the Night-Before-an-Event Plate? We know from scientific studies that you want to top off your glycogen stores before a big event. That is, you need to fill your tank with slow-acting carbohydrates the day before, so when you perform the next day, you don't hit the wall and have your body use protein or fat for energy. The Night-Before-an-Event Plate adjusts the Healthy Plate to add more of these slow-acting carbohydrates than protein.

I devised the Night-Before-an-Event Plate over time from seeing people eat all that pasta before road races. Research presented at sports medicine meetings shows you need to eat protein, not eliminate it, the night before an event. Not only will this fuel your body for the event, it will help you have a healthier and quicker recovery from post-event muscle soreness. This comes from microtears in muscles during extensive exercise. You need the amino acids from protein on board to be ready to repair muscles. The more you have available in your body, the better prepared it will be to prevent post-event muscle soreness.

NIGHT-BEFORE-AN-EVENT PLATE

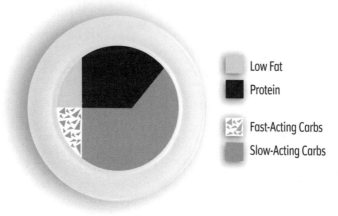

Low Fat

Protein

Fast-Acting Carbs

Slow-Acting Carbs

The Night-Before-an-Event Plate cuts down a little on protein, which the body needs to break down into amino acids during exercise. Too much protein may make you feel the way you do on Thanksgiving Day if you eat too much turkey: the protein in the turkey makes you feel tired the next day.

You will get fast-acting carbohydrates in the morning of the event, for example, from an "Elvis bagel." I have seen athletes use up their body's stored fuel just by nervous energy before an event. If you lie awake worrying about the event the next day, you may not get a good night's sleep and end up burning fuel stores. If you have some fast-acting carbohydrates on board by eating them in the morning, you will have the sugar you need to fuel the beginning of the event and not have to go into your body's glycogen stores too soon.

"Carbo Loading" and Pasta Parties

I spoke at the Leukemia & Lymphoma Society's Team in Training dinner before the New York City Marathon and told the runners, I see you think this is your last meal. It's not. You will make it through the marathon tomorrow. Put a little chicken on your plate to go with your pasta, and you will see you will feel better and maybe even run faster tomorrow.

After the race, Jeff, a fit sixty-year-old accountant, came up to me. "Doc, you were so right. I cut down on the amount of pasta I would normally eat before a race and added in some chicken breasts. I felt much stronger during the race. Actually, the difference was remarkable. I've been running for twenty years. I just set my personal best by more than ten minutes."

Pasta parties, where runners gather together and everyone eats plates and plates of pasta, used to be all the rage. It became a marathon tradition the night before to "carbo load." In fact, the New York City Marathon used to be sponsored by Ronzoni, the pasta manufacturer, and the Barilla (another pasta manufacturer) Marathon Eve Dinner fed 15,000 marathoners and their guests 6,840 pounds of pasta. This was based on the ill-conceived concept of loading up on carbohydrates. Then sports medicine studies revealed more information about how to prepare your body for such an event and found runners needed protein as well.

Some running organizations who put on big races and charity events still organize a pasta buffet, which is now more of a smorgasbord. If you go to one of these eating events, make sure to put some chicken, meat, or a large helping of cheese on your plate for protein.

Another mistake is to think this will be your last meal. Do not go back for two or three plates of food. If you eat too much pasta the night before an event, this may cause you to need to go to the bathroom during the event. Tennis players may need a bathroom break in between sets if they eat too much the night before. I've seen marathon runners have to dash between cars on the streets of New York to urgently relieve themselves.

The most recent scientific evidence states the vertical part of your Night-Before-an-Event Plate shouldn't be more than normal. If you have been eating the Healthy Plate, just make the adjustments I suggested above for the Night-Before-an-Event Plate. This is a specialized situation that just needs a little tweaking.

Timing

If you normally eat at, say, 6:30 PM before an event, keep the same schedule. I've been at pasta parties that go on well past 9:00 PM. This change in your eating habit will not help you perform better. When you eat later in the night, food will still be digesting and lying in your stomach when you go to bed, and you may not sleep well. You may also end up needing to move your bowels during the event. If you normally eat later, eat at an earlier time so your body is ready for the race the next day.

If your timing is off, including your food intake, your performance may be off, too. Do nothing new to prepare for the day of an event. That includes the timing of *when* you eat as well as *what* you eat.

Drinking

I highly recommend you stay away from caffeine the night before an event. Caffeine can dehydrate you. Watch your urine color to make sure you are not drinking too much or too little liquid the day and night before an event. Also, if you increase your caffeine intake too much, this can make your heart susceptible to sudden death (see Chapter 15).

Stay away from too much alcohol. Alcohol makes you sleepy and may throw off your sleep cycle. It may also dehydrate you. If you usually drink a glass a wine with dinner, that's okay; don't change your drinking habit.

Drawing the Night-Before-an-Event Plate

Over the last few years, I have begun to draw out the Night-Before-an-Event Plate to show my patients how to use it. I draw the plate on the paper on the examination table, and then we discuss it. I tell them what to put on the plate and have them visualize what to eat. They easily get the idea. It's simple and it works. They are eating healthy for the event without even thinking about it. When I talk at pre-event dinners, I show the Healthy Plate and then the Night-Before-an-Event Plate. Thousands of people have learned about how to use the Night-Before-an-Event Plate to perform at their best.

When choosing the foods for your Night-Before-an-Event Plate, remember to choose the freshest, most colorful produce. With the game you played by buying different color produce, you should have a better idea of what to look for. You can tell the difference between healthy and not-so-healthy foods by their color. To add protein to your Night-Before-an-Event Plate, choose meat that is bright red, not brown, in color. Like an artist who paints with acrylics, you have hundreds of shades of foods to choose from. When you shop in a market, look at the multitudes of colors of food, and choose the brightest for the most concentrated nutrients.

The bottom-line message is: don't get caught in the fanfare or circus that goes on before a race or any big event, for example, a tennis or golf tournament. This also applies even to a 10K race or your long run of the week. Follow the same precepts outlined above about what to eat and drink. Stick with your plan. Do nothing new the night before an event. If you go to a pre-event party, be mindful about what you eat at the buffet. Only you are responsible for what you eat. The party may be lots of fun with your friends and guest speakers, but be careful about how you fuel yourself in order to perform and feel your best the next day.

The way you prepare before an event helps during race day. The next chapter reveals how to fuel yourself after a long event to recover faster.

CHAPTER NINE

The After-a-Long-Workout Plate

Mac, a fifty-two-year-old businessman, came in to see me the day after running his very first New York City Marathon. He joined the long line of patients in my waiting room. Most of them were first-time marathon runners who came in with sore muscles.

"I have never felt this sore in my life after a race," said Mac, who had played tennis and volleyball in college. "I'm really scared that something is very wrong with me." I explained what he was feeling was post-event soreness due to inflammation of muscles. I recommended he apply ice on the sore areas, using a Ziploc freezer bag filled with a combination of ice and water, and I suggested he get a sports massage. Since Mac had no kidney or heart problems, I told him to take two non-steroidal anti-inflammatory agents over the next few days to help ease the muscle pain.

I also outlined the After-a-Long-Workout Plate and gave him some tips on how to prevent muscle soreness. Mac said later, "I learned from the experience. For my next tennis tournament, I used the After-a-Long-Workout Plate afterwards, plus icing and NSAIDs, and I was only sore for one day. I knew what to do and what to eat, and it helped."

After a long workout or a strenuous event such as a race, artificial recovery drinks don't cut it. These specialized sports drinks are mostly sugar and salt, with no protein, and therefore don't allow you to repair your muscles. This chapter reviews the best recovery drink (hint: you probably drank it as a kid) and how to fill out the After-a-Long-Workout Plate.

In order to understand what to eat and drink, you need to understand what you are "recovering" from. When you exercise, muscle membrane breaks down on a microscopic level, and there are microtears of muscles, tendons, and ligaments. Healing and minimizing post-event muscle soreness depends on having amino acids in your body to rebuild the protein in these structures. You should also replenish the carbohydrates and fats that were used to provide energy during your race or long workout. Therefore, a good diet all week that includes the basic food groups, using the Healthy Plate and Training Plate, is important.

The After-a-Long-Workout Plate contains more fat and more fast-acting carbohydrates than the other Fueling Plates. The After-a-Long-Workout Plate has a higher percentage of fat than the other Fueling Plates because you need energy to rebound. Fat is a good source of energy now, the kind of energy to get you moving again. After a long workout, fast-acting carbohydrates are used up by the initial burst of energy, as are most of your glycogen stores from slow-acting carbohydrates. To feel better afterward, you need a good amount of protein (though not as much as for the Healthy Plate or Training Plate), which breaks down to amino acids ready to be available to repair muscles in the next day or two.

AFTER-A-LONG-WORKOUT PLATE

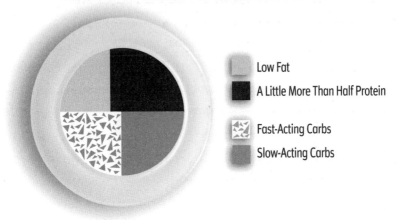

Low Fat

A Little More Than Half Protein

Fast-Acting Carbs

Slow-Acting Carbs

Five Points to Remember After a Long Workout or Event

The goals after a long workout or event are to: replenish your glycogen; give you back some energy because you are tired; provide protein for amino acids to build muscles; drink liquids to rehydrate; and help decrease the time of post-event soreness.

These five points are easy to accomplish. Here's how to do it:

Replenish your glycogen. You likely have used up your glycogen stores during the long event. It's like refilling your gas tank, which is probably down to one-eighth. The post-event meal is your gas station to fill up your fuel tank. The best way to do that is to eat foods proportionally using the After-a-Long-Workout Plate.

Restore energy. Most people are tired after a long workout. To build back protein from amino acids requires energy. Fats are a good source of energy because during extended exercise you likely have used up some fat stores. You can use some fatty acids and some fast-acting carbohydrates to provide that energy.

Provide protein to build muscles. The After-a-Long-Workout Plate has some protein because you need more protein after a long event. It does not contain as much protein as the Training Plate, but almost as much. Microtears need amino acids on board to rebuild muscles. Do it now by eating some protein to get that process going.

Rehydrate. After a long workout, the best drink is plain old water. Don't down sports drinks right after a long exercise bout until you have checked your urine. The kidneys eliminate salt from the body through urine and retain water up to thirty minutes after you have stopped exercising. If you pop two non-steroidal anti-inflammatory drug (NSAID) pills after an event for muscle soreness, all you do is maintain fluid in the kidneys, and you can become hyponatremic. Take NSAIDs after you are eating, drinking, and urinating normally. Checking your urine is most important. If you sweated a lot during exercise and your urine looks dark, like the color of iced tea, drink more. You need to stay well hydrated after extensive exercise. You may feel sluggish if you are not properly hydrated, and your body's repair mechanism may slow down. As we discussed earlier in the book, drink enough so that your urine is the color of lemonade.

Reduce post-event soreness. You want to minimize the likelihood and the amount of post-event soreness. Eating the right foods will play a large role in the recovery of your muscles, as well as some other techniques, such as icing and using NSAIDs.

Massage

The day after a long event, your muscles may ache, particularly if you did not have enough protein before or after the event. Perhaps you took a hot shower right afterward, and this caused even more muscle inflammation and pain.

The day after the event is a good time to get a massage, but not immediately afterward. Lactic acid builds up after a long workout. Some massage therapists claim within an hour of an event they get lactic acid out of muscles with a massage, but they really are just moving the lactic acid around and making more microtears, the byproduct of exercise. The day after the event is the best time for a sports massage to help move lactic acid out of muscles and into the blood circulation to help neutralize it.

After a long workout, I suggest you take a cool shower. A hot shower inflames muscles. Or, if you are really sore, try an ice bath. If you are still in pain for five to seven days after the long workout, you won't want to go back and do it again. The goal is to recover quickly, so you do want to repeat a similar long event in the future.

Timing

When should you eat after a long workout? The answer is after you have rehydrated enough so that your urine is normal. When you perform a long workout, you may retain fluid. Until your urine is normal color, hold off on eating, usually about thirty minutes. After any endurance exercise, blood is redirected to limbs that were active. You need time for the blood flow to be redirected to the gut before you start eating. Otherwise, you may feel nauseous if you eat right away.

As I cautioned in the Night Before-an-Event Plate, the first meal after a long workout is not your last meal. If you eat too much by going too vertical on the After-a-Long-Workout Plate, you may feel bloated. With some practice, you will know how high to pile the food in the four sections of the After-a-Long-Workout Plate. Use your experience with this plate to put the right quantity of fast-acting carbohydrates, slow-acting carbohydrates, protein, and fat on your plate to prevent post-event muscle soreness.

Low-Fat Chocolate Milk

Some artificial recovery drinks have protein, but most have none. The best recovery drink is low-fat chocolate milk—it has protein in the milk and sugar in the chocolate, and it is low in fat. There's not too much fat to affect your coronary arteries, some sugar for immediate energy recovery, and protein from the milk to help build back microtears in muscles.

Chocolate milk has nine essential nutrients, including calcium, potassium, and vitamin D. New research implies there are antioxidant properties in cocoa and chocolate milk, so it may be good for your heart. No other single beverage replaces the nutrient-rich package found in milk. Low-fat or skim chocolate milk has a valuable role in the diet as a way of increasing consumption by palatability and taste. If you can't drink milk due to lactose intolerance, you can use a sports drink designed with some of the same ingredients.

After a hard workout, if you do decide to have a recovery drink, make sure that it has carbohydrates as well as added protein in a 3:1 or 4:1 ratio of carbohydrates to protein so that you have amino acids available for muscle repair. I prefer that you do not choose a recovery drink, but instead eat protein in your next meal. Along with chocolate milk, peanut butter and jelly sandwiches, pretzels and cheese, and fortified tomato juice are all good food alternatives to recovery drinks. Many runners I know love french fries and chocolate milk after a marathon—it works great and you deserve the treat!

If you do all of the above, you should recover quickly and feel great.

Beer

A number of road races now have beer gardens available to participants after the race. Why drink beer? Some sports science research studies now suggest that drinking a beer after running a 10K or longer event reverses the "marathon kidney" physiology that changes the way the body handles salt and sets up hyponatremia. That is, the alcohol in beer appears to normalize kidney function.

Nutritionally, beer has carbohydrates, which are good after a long workout. You might want to also have a knockwurst for some fat and protein. Just drinking beer after a long event is like just eating pasta beforehand and is not recommended. Again, make sure you are properly hydrated and your urine is the right color before drinking beer. Beer actually does have some medicinal purposes, in combination with a fatty food, and in moderation, obviously.

My final message for this chapter is if you are smart about what you do after a long workout, you will feel better and will recover quicker.

In the next chapter, we will examine how to use Fueling Plates at Home and Away.

CHAPTER TEN

Fueling Plates at Home and Away

When I met Tim, then a fifty-year-old builder, he said he ran to prevent a heart attack because his father died of a heart attack at age fifty-two. "I average sixty miles a week and run four marathons a year. I feel like I have to run. I'm afraid of dying at a young age," said Tim. "My doctor wanted to put me on a statin to reduce my cholesterol level, but I told him I'll just run more."

Tim's doctor also suggested he lose five to ten pounds to get to his ideal body weight and reduce his heart disease risk. "I have tried every diet, and I watch what I eat. What am I supposed to do, carry a scale around with me?" he asked.

I showed Tim how to use the Healthy Plate at home and when he goes out to eat. He went through the four-week Fueling Plates program, checking in with me once a week to show me what he was eating and how he was doing. When he was training for a long run, he used the Training Plate.

"I continued using the Healthy Plate and Training Plate, and after eight weeks, my total cholesterol was down to 200 from 270 and I had lost *four pounds. Using the Healthy Plate was easy, but more importantly, I was losing weight slowly. I've gone to nutritionists and read countless diet books. Nobody made it this simple," said Tim. In another two months, Tim had lost another four pounds.*

"Now I'm fifty-five and have lived longer than my father. I lost the weight I needed to and have kept the weight off. I learned how to move things around on my plate and to ask for an extra plate at restaurants to take food home with me. Food still tastes good, and I feel better than I ever have," said Tim.

*I*t's easy to make use of the Fueling Plates program at home because you have cooked the foods yourself. You simply divide the plate into the appropriate amounts of the four basic food groups—slow-acting carbohydrates, fast-acting carbohydrates, protein, and fat—as described in earlier chapters. When you are away from home, you have to be like a kid playing with your food.

This chapter explains how to make use of the Fueling Plates at home, for you and your family, and at a restaurant, to divide the food up on your plate as you would at home. In that way you won't overeat one food group and undereat another food group.

At Home

At home, with a little practice, it's relatively easy to learn how to use the Fueling Plates program. If you find you have a problem visualizing where the four basic food groups should go on your plate, you can practice using whatever Fueling Plate you choose. Look up the appropriate Fueling Plate diagram in this book and mark up a paper plate with the four sections to match it. Now put your food into the appropriate sections and really look at how the food looks on the plate. Make a mental picture. You now know how the ingredients of this dish fit into the Fueling Plate.

I recommend you take a copy of the Healthy Plate sheet with you when you go to the market. Pick out a chicken dinner based on what will fit on the Healthy Plate. For example, my favorite chicken dinner is "Cornflake Chicken." I dip the chicken breasts in a small amount of healthy oil (such as extra virgin olive oil), coat the chicken with crumbled corn flakes (plain, not sugar-coated), and bake at 350°F for forty-five minutes.

The chicken is, of course, the protein. The corn flakes are a fast- to medium-acting carbohydrate. To get in some slow-acting carbohydrates, I add in a side dish of steamed green beans and mushrooms. Or I may add in some mashed potatoes (fast-acting carbohydrate) and low-fat milk (protein). If I need more fat, I'll put a pat of butter on the green beans. If I need more slow-acting carbohydrates, I make some whole-grain rice.

Depending on which plate I'm using, I can adjust this basic recipe with side dishes to fill up the appropriate sections of the Fueling Plate. This is a simple way to fill any of the Fueling Plates at home.

Another plus to eating this way instead of a restrictive fad diet is that you can make the same meal for your whole family—and you will all benefit from eating healthily with the Fueling Plates program. You know if it fills up the Healthy Plate, it will be a healthy meal. Don't just serve your child a plate of macaroni and cheese, which has a lot fat; add in some vegetables, too. Even young kids can use the Healthy Plate, and they may help you see how much fun it can be to move food around on the plate. Do well for yourself and make the same dinner for you and your entire family. Everyone will feel better.

Away

Sarah, a twenty-three-year-old social worker, had used the Fueling Plates program for two months but felt embarrassed to move the food around on her plate when she went to a restaurant. "I used the program to eat more healthy foods, and I was feeling good about it, but I was reluctant to use the plates away from home. Then I went to my favorite fish place with some friends and was served an absolutely beautiful portion of salmon, but it was huge. I knew I couldn't eat it all, so I asked the waiter for an extra plate," said Sarah. "I told my friends about the Fueling Plates program and showed them how to move the food into four sections of the plate. By the time we had finished the meal, everyone else at the table had also asked for a second plate to take some food home. We were having fun with it.

"Now when I go out to eat, I still do the Fueling Plates program," said Sarah. "It's more exciting because when I go to a restaurant, I can look at the offerings of side dishes and fill up my plate as if I was at a smorgasbord to make sure I get in all four food groups. I make a game of it."

I have to admit that top chefs hate me when I take apart their beautifully prepared food at a fancy restaurant. But I always take a photo of the dish first and post it on Facebook before I mess it up. I know how much time and effort it takes to prepare food served in such a beautiful, artistic manner.

When out at a restaurant, I like to order roast chicken on a plate of leeks or mashed potatoes. I put the chicken in the protein area of my Healthy Plate. The leeks are slow-acting carbohydrates, and the potatoes I put into the fast-acting carbohydrate area. The sauce on top of the chicken is my fat. I visualize the amount of fat from the sauce, and realize I don't need any more fat. I may also order a side dish of steamed asparagus or peas and carrots. If there's too much food, I fill a second plate with the extra food and ask the waiter to box it up to go. I make sure the proportions are the same in the boxed-up food so I know I have the makings of another Healthy Plate when I'm back home.

My friend Tom Keller, the chef/owner of the restaurant Per Se, serves dishes filled mostly with protein. He believes in the Healthy Plate because it affords you the opportunity to order sides and fill out the plate. When you go to a nice restaurant, like Per Se, take a look at the menu and ask your server exactly what is in the dish you are considering. In particular, ask what is served with the protein, so you can fill up your Healthy Plate with appropriate side dishes.

Start to visualize your Healthy Plate as you read the menu. Let's say you're looking at the pork chop. Okay, this is your protein. You need a slow-acting carbohydrate, so consider ordering string beans almandine, which has slow-acting carbohydrates in the beans and some nuts for additional protein. Or maybe you are in the mood for mashed yams and its slow-acting carbohydrates. The pork chop comes with applesauce, so there's the fast-acting carbohydrate. The sauce on the pork chop likely has some fat in it. If you think you need more fat, add a pat of butter to the beans or yams.

It's often hard to know where the fat is in a dish, but it's likely in the sauce. You can live with a little more fat for one night, even if it's a so-called "bad" fat. At your next meal at home, use more healthy fats. You're allowed to treat yourself every once in a while, just not every day. If you get the slow-acting carbohydrates, fast-acting carbohydrates, and protein down when you eat out, the fat will come your way. But don't order fried chicken, thinking you need lots of fat. If you are using the Healthy Plate all the time, you can have some fried or sautéed foods, which might have a little more fat.

You can even go to a bar and order platters of pub food that would likely fill you up for days if you ate it all. Here's the challenge: when the waiter brings you so much food, you need to pick out the foods that fit into the Healthy Plate. For example, if you order a pu pu platter, choose the spare ribs, but you don't also have to eat the fried wontons. Order a side salad (no cheese fries!). Once you start thinking about the Fueling Plates and make it part of your routine, you will have a different perspective on how to order food when you go out. You'll be pleasantly surprised at how simple it is to eat out and eat healthily.

To make it easier for you to choose, take the illustrations of Fueling Plates from this book with you—either a printed copy or a picture on your phone—and consult them when you order. When you're out at dinner, you can peruse the illustrations and then separate out the food on your plate to fit whatever Fueling Plate you are using.

In a way, it's easier to use the Fueling Plates program away from home because you don't have so many steps; for example, planning your menu and then going to the market and picking out the food. At the restaurant, you can just look at the menu and order. The disadvantage is that some of the process is out of your hands. When you are home, you choose your own food, and you know *exactly* what you're getting. If I pick out a zucchini at the market, I know I will get the freshest one with the most micronutrients possible. In a restaurant, I am relying on the chef to pick healthy ingredients. However, most good chefs have lots of experience picking out the tastiest vegetables at the market.

To sum up, when you're eating out, it's pretty much the same as at home in terms of using the Fueling Plates; you just have to play the game slightly differently. At home, you decide what to put on your plate depending on which Fueling Plate you are using and pick out the food to fill up the plate. When you go out, you have to come at the Fueling Plate from a different angle. With the menu in front of you, first visualize the plate and pick out the foods to put on the plate. Don't be intimidated about making reasonable special requests. Check out how the food will be cooked and tell the waiter how you prefer it, for example, steamed, not sautéed vegetables. If the serving size is too large, which is likely in today's restaurant world, ask for a second plate and box and take home the food on the second plate with you as leftovers.

Next, we examine how to use the Fueling Plates program to lose or gain weight.

CHAPTER ELEVEN

Fueling Plates to Lose Weight and Gain Weight

*T*his chapter details how to use the Fueling Plates to lose or gain weight. To lose weight, eat a little less of the four basic food groups, using the Training Plate. You are going to get enough good food to feel good as you continue training. To gain weight, do the opposite: add a little more height to your Training Plate. You don't need to go overboard, just add slightly more food to each of the four sections of the plate.

Is that enough? Yes, just adjust the height of the slow-acting carbohydrates, fact-acting carbohydrates, protein, and fat. In order to lose or gain weight and stay healthy, just increase or decrease the vertical height of these food groups. Many people think the only way to lose weight is to stop eating certain foods, to eat only a specialized diet, or decrease the number of calories they eat. I don't like using the term "calories" because then you have to count them. I prefer you just lower the height to lose weight or raise the height to gain weight.

Exercise, a Key Component

Nancy, a forty-five-year-old secretary, had volunteered to participate in a Leukemia & Lymphoma 10K event to raise money for her friend who had just been diagnosed with acute myeloid leukemia. She came to see me to prepare for the race. "Look at me; I look fat. I eat the right food, I follow the recommendation to get on the scale every day, but I don't lose weight. Sometimes I starve myself, and then I eat too much," said Nancy.

We discussed the Training Plate. I showed her how to use it to train for the upcoming race and also to lose some weight. "I decreased the proportions of the foods I was eating using the Training Plate and began a walking program. I used my cell phone to make sure I got in 10,000 steps each day," said Nancy. "Then I started to jog a little and walk some, then run some more and walk less. I had never run before."

After two months of training, Nancy had lost four pounds. She completed the 10K race, alternating running and walking. "I was hooked. Within a year, I trained for a half-marathon and lost twenty-five pounds by upping my exercise intensity. Then I trained for a full marathon. It took me four and a half hours to complete. Before I had lost the weight, it probably would have taken me six and a half hours. I'm ecstatic about losing the weight!" said Nancy.

For most people, eating less or more is not enough to lose or gain weight, respectively. Exercise is a key component to losing or gaining weight. If you haven't begun a routine exercise program, now is the time to do that. Start slowly by simply walking. Use your cell phone or a wristwatch device to count your steps and work your way up to 10,000 steps a day. No one knows how many steps are correct for you, but most doctors use this number as a good benchmark of daily steps. Don't get discouraged if you don't hit your goal right away; just keep at it.

Exercise is important because, if you want to lose weight, you need to increase the set point of your metabolism. The control of your body weight appears to be similar to a set point, relying upon an internal body fat thermostat that is sensitive to total body fat and has the ability to influence a range of responses to increase total body fat (eating more food, reducing metabolic rate) or decrease total body fat (eating less food, increasing metabolic rate). This set-point theory is not completely understood, but studies show it relies, in part, upon hormones, such as leptin and insulin, which are released into the blood in proportion to body fat and influence specific brain centers controlling food intake.

One way to influence your metabolic set point is through aerobic exercise. You can reset the metabolic set point higher with regular exercise. That's why diet alone is often not enough to sustain weight loss.

If you want to gain weight, the Training Plate is also a great tool to accompany an exercise program. It can help you make sure you get an adequate amount of protein while you exercise. As you increase the intensity of your training, you may need to slightly increase the height of the protein portion on your plate, which is exactly what you do with the Training Plate. You need the protein to make sure the extra food you eat does not turn into fat. Instead, as you train, the extra protein will lead to increased muscle mass and increase your weight.

Losing Weight

To lose weight, eat a little less of everything on the Training Plate than it takes to feel as if your belly is full. Walk away from the table slightly hungry. Since everyone's metabolism is different, rather than measuring out your food or counting calories, as in popular diet programs, just use hunger as a guide. Also, drink more water than normal.

The best way to lose weight is to combine diet and exercise. If you really want to lose the fat weight, you need to increase muscle mass to be toned. By doing aerobic exercise, you will increase your metabolic set point so you can eat more food without gaining weight.

The newest recommendations are to do some aerobic exercise every day. This could be to count your steps to get in at least 10,000 steps a day, or make sure you do some aerobic exercise for twenty minutes at a time, three times a week. As I mentioned, start slowly if need be and work your way up to 10,000 steps, or begin with ten minutes of aerobic exercise daily and work up to twenty minutes a day. And it doesn't have to be twenty minutes all at once. New research shows even a few minutes of intense exercise several times a day can help you meet this exercise requirement.

Don't forget strength training. Even runners who run six days a week need to go to the gym to do some strength training. If you need help devising a muscle-strengthening program, ask a trainer at your local gym to help set you up with a circuit. Aim for one hour of a full-body workout, three times a week. Sports science studies show you need to work out three times a week to get in enough repetitions to gain muscle mass and strength.

Or you can do the lower body one day—hips, buttocks, legs, and calves—and upper body another day—neck, shoulders, arms, back, and abdomen. Remain active on the days in between the workouts.

Obligate Runner

I know people who are what psychiatrist Alayne Yates and her colleagues at the University of Arizona Health Sciences Center refer to as the "obligate runner." These people run compulsively. If they eat a slice of pizza, they go out and run a few extra miles afterward to "work it off." They have a drive that preempts fulfillment in other life areas or may run to the point of inflicting physical damage on their bodies. Up to one-quarter of serious runners may be neurotically attached to their sport.

Usually, the obligate runner takes up serious running—defined as more than forty miles per week—relatively late in life as compared to other athletes. Obligate runners often feel unfulfilled in their professional or personal lives, and use running as a method for achieving meaning. They may also use running as an aid toward denying aging, physical dissolution, and death.

Running can be very fulfilling and a way to stay healthy. But if you get too obsessed with running, you may lose sight of the rest of your life. You may lose weight through running, but are you truly happy? Keep your exercise in perspective and be like a bee—look for the honey in the moments of your life.

Gaining Weight

Alex, a forty-year-old account executive, wanted to gain weight to look better. He was compulsive about his work. "I go to work at 8 AM and get home at 10 PM. I barely have time to eat," said Alex.

We discussed the Training Plate and his need to increase the height on the plate to gain weight. I suggested he go to the gym in his office building at lunch hour every day, and then eat a protein-packed lunch at his desk. The other two days, I suggested he walk for twenty minutes on a path near his building before lunch.

"I asked the trainer in my gym to show me how to use the weight machines, and he gave a few different workouts. I slowly added more weight each week. I gained fifteen pounds in one year. That's exactly what I wanted to do. Now I fill out my suits. As an added benefit, I made some new friends at the gym and joined the pickup basketball game," said Alex.

The purpose of gaining weight is to increase your muscle mass. You need to eat more in proportion to what's on your Training Plate but with a higher level of each of the food groups, protein in particular.

You don't want to gain weight by gaining fat. If you eat too many carbohydrates and fat each day, you will gain fat. Instead, eat the same amounts on the Training Plate, but more of it at each meal. The Training Plate has more protein than the other Fueling Plates, so you will automatically increase the protein portion of the food you eat.

Some athletes use creatine to help them gain muscle mass. It can work to bulk you up if you follow the directions on the label. But I have found that you may get injured more frequently if you use creatine. Muscle pulls and tears are more common in those athletes who take creatine, and I don't recommend it.

My strong suggestion is to build up your muscles in the gym by doing heavier strength-training workouts. Do a full-body weight workout and increase the weight of each exercise by a maximum of 10 percent per week. As the weight increases, your muscles will increase, and your body weight will increase, too. By doing increased weight training and by eating in the right proportion, you won't increase fat, but you will increase muscle mass.

Remember to also do aerobic exercise as well, even if only walking for twenty minutes at a time, three times a week, at a minimum. A lot of athletes who want to gain weight, such as weight lifters, tend not to do aerobic exercise.

Set SMART Goals

If you're looking to lose weight or gain weight, the first step is to set yourself a goal. Set a goal you can accomplish. Short-term goals are better than long-term ones. If you want to run a marathon, you need to take baby steps and run a 5K, a 10K, and then a half-marathon before you get to a full marathon. It's the same with weight loss or weight gain. Small steps, a pound or two at a time, are what you are looking for.

To lose weight, gain weight, or make any changes in your health, you need to set SMART goals. SMART is an acronym for Specific, Measurable, Attainable, Relevant, and Timely. This will help you set and enact your goals.

Specific: Define the goal as much as possible with no ambiguous language. Know who is involved, what you want to accomplish, where it will be done, your reasons for making the change, and any constraints or requirements you may have.

Measurable: Can you track your progress and measure the outcome? How will you know when you have accomplished your goal?

Attainable: Is the goal reasonable enough to be accomplished? Make sure the goal is not out of reach.

Relevant: Is the goal worthwhile, and will it meet your needs? Is the goal consistent with other goals you have established, and does it fit with your intermediate and long-term plans?

Timely: Set a time limit, say, thirty days. This will establish a sense of urgency and prompt you to have better time management.

Are you ready to change your mindset? Start small, slow, and make gradual progress. Stay focused. Prepare for barriers, such as lapses and setbacks. Remain positive—pick yourself up and get back on track if you do fall back into bad habits. There is no diet that will do what healthy eating does. Skip the diet and just eat healthily by using the Training Plate.

In conclusion, to lose or gain weight, first choose baby-step changes, use the Training Plate, and then tweak your plan to meet your goals. Know the reason for the tweaking, and you will end up reaching your goal. Learn how to use the Training Plate to your advantage. I can't emphasize enough that losing weight or gaining weight is not purely about what's on your plate. Remember to exercise, and you will meet and maintain your weight goals.

Next, we will introduce the best sports-specific nutrition guidelines for a multitude of sports.

CHAPTER TWELVE

Sports-Specific Nutrition

*E*very athlete strives for an edge over his or her competition. A comprehensive eating plan, such as the Fueling Plates program, complements daily training and recovery to help you meet these physical demands. The key is to achieve peak nutritional performance to aid your training and let you compete at your best.

This chapter provides an overview of sports-specific nutrition guidelines, which you can adapt to your individual needs based on the distinct characteristics of each sport. Off-season workouts and training programs may require different considerations, based on the nature and goals of your off-season program. For example, your energy requirements may be much higher as you begin training for an event. During this period, building in time for recovery is important. Or you may be looking to lose fat and gain lean mass, which would require a slightly different nutrition strategy (see Chapter 11). The recommendations in this chapter focus on your nutrition needs during regular exercise and training for competition.

I can't tell you how many times I have patients who come to see me say, "I'm not an athlete." When I ask them what they do for exercise, I hear, "I run twenty-five miles a week" or "I play in two soccer leagues, one on a weeknight, the other on the weekend, and work out at the gym." Who wouldn't say those people are not athletes? With all the professional and college sports now available 24–7 on television and the Internet, everyday people often look down on what they do as not being "athletic."

If you engage in regular activity up to three hours a week, then consider yourself a recreational athlete. If you exercise for three to six hours a week, then you are a competitive athlete. You may not need the same amount of nutrition as a professional athlete, who usually exercises more than six hours a week, but the sports-specific foods you need are basically the same.

Recreational Athlete

Good nutrition can enhance the sporting performance of recreational athletes. A well-planned, nutritious diet should meet most of your vitamin and mineral needs, and provide enough protein to promote muscle growth and repair. Foods rich in slow-acting, unrefined carbohydrates, like whole-grain breads and cereals, should form the basis of the diet, which is what you get when you follow the Healthy Plate. Water is a great choice of fluid for all athletes to help performance and prevent dehydration.

Basic nutrition from a healthy, balanced diet (the Healthy Plate) is all the recreational athlete needs. On training days, you need slightly more nutrients and fluids because you will expend more energy. This calls for the Training Plate. For exercise that goes on for less than one hour, water is sufficient to cover your fluid requirements. If your exercise lasts longer than one hour, use a sports drink. And remember to drink more fluids before and after sport activities.

Competitive Athlete

A basic nutrition plan (again, the Healthy Plate) is just as fundamental for the competitive athlete. In addition, when you plan to compete, you will likely require more energy in the form of long-acting carbohydrates and protein. The fluid recommendations are the same as the recreational athlete. If the exertion is shorter than one hour, water is enough; for more than one hour, use a sports drink.

Competition or longer exercise bouts require more carbohydrates. Carbohydrate stores are depleted after about one hour of an intensive workout. Everyone's metabolism is different, so it's difficult to say what your optimal requirements are or when to add carbohydrates during a workout to replenish any depleted fuel stores and restore muscle glycogen. Here are some general guidelines on how much carbohydrates you may need after exercise:

- Less than forty-five minutes of activity: no carbohydrates needed.
- Forty-five minutes to seventy-five minutes of activity: small amount of carbohydrates needed. A mouth rinse of a sports drink will do.
- One to two hours of activity: 30 grams of carbohydrates per hour. Two-thirds of a cup of long-grain rice.
- Two to three hours of activity: 60 grams of carbohydrates per hour. Two large bananas.
- More than three hours of activity: 90 grams of carbohydrates per hour. A plate of pasta and two slices of bread.

You can see you don't need large amounts of carbohydrates to perform. It all depends on how long you are active. You may need just a mouth rinse of a sports drink, or something a lot more.

Nutrition and Fluid Needs for Specific Sports

Good nutrition and hydration practices are two important components to successful individual performance. Every sport is different, and factors such as rules of play, frequency of games, length of season, and position-specific requirements may alter your nutritional plans. The characteristics of the sports may vary—one sport may be "stop and go" with high-intensity bursts followed by lower intensity or rest periods, such as tennis, while another may be repetitive, constant motion, such as running a long road race. No matter the sport, you need to know what's best to eat or drink on top of the Healthy Plate or Training Plate.

Here's a rundown, sport-by-sport, of training, nutrition, and fluid requirements.

Baseball and Softball

Baseball is primarily a sprint rather than an endurance sport. The longest you will have to run is 360 feet, slightly more than 100 yards, when legging out an inside-the-park home run. In between pitches and waiting to bat, you do a lot of standing around or sitting in the dugout. But when the time comes, you have to run in short sprints.

Even though they know that baseball requires fast bursts, most baseball players don't condition themselves well. Softball players are even worse off since many do not even consider themselves athletes.

Baseball and softball players have lower overall energy demands during games, but they spend many hours on the playing field during summer months. Hydration can become a concern in the heat. Also, make sure your blood sugar levels are adequate during games to keep your mind and body sharp to make decisions on the ball field. I recommend homemade gorp with low-fat granola, raisins or dried cranberries, nibs of dark chocolate, and salted mixed nuts.

Basketball

Like other running sports, basketball requires superb conditioning. You must be able to exert a burst of speed to get by the person guarding you and also have the endurance to run the court for an entire game. If you play in pickup games, you may play several games over the course of a day. You also need to develop a good first step and side-to-side agility.

For these short, fast-acting motions plus endurance, maintain yourself with the Healthy Plate. The main issue is before game day. Make sure to eat an "Elvis bagel," my version of Elvis Presley's favorite breakfast—a bagel for slow-acting carbohydrates, a banana for fast-acting carbohydrates, and peanut butter for protein and a little fat—or the equivalent, such as an English muffin, fried egg, and jelly or a biscuit with scrambled eggs and jam.

Eat two hours before game time. I suggest a cocktail of fresh fruits, such as apples and berries. Fructose is a natural sugar that is broken down to blood sugars that are maintained in the body more than just simple sugar. This will help you last longer during the game. Between two hours and game time, check your urine for hydration and drink more fluids, if need be. Refrain from eating anything right before the game. Also, have more fruit available for half time, such as cut-up oranges.

Cycling

To increase your cycling efficiency, you should work on your leg strength first and foremost, since this is your means of locomotion.

Cycling also calls for strong buttock muscles as well as solid calves for pedaling.

Good nutrition for cyclists means replacing the nutrients you lost during your workout. In response to your ride, your appetite will likely increase above the level you are used to as your body releases hunger hormones in its mission to maintain body fat stores. If you are using the Healthy Plate in general or the Training Plate before a race, you are getting the slow-acting carbohydrates, fast-acting carbohydrates, protein, good fats, and vitamins and minerals you need. Time your pre-ride meal for at least ninety minutes prior to hitting the road. Make sure you drink enough during your ride—carry a water bottle with you.

Your exercise intensity and how long you ride will dictate whether you need to eat anything during the ride. Solid foods, such as energy bars, are usually better tolerated toward the beginning of a ride and are ideal to take about halfway through a long ride. Some of these bars may be hard to digest, so practice with them first before using them during a high-intensity race, and drink plenty of water along with them.

Football

The most important thing a football player can do is improve conditioning. Statistics show that injuries tend to occur at the end of a half because players are fatigued. Proper warm-up, cool-down, and flexibility exercises can help you avoid muscle pulls. Cool down and stretch after exercising to avoid soreness and stiffness the next day. Weekend football players need total body stretching but should concentrate on the lower body, which is where most muscle pulls in football occur.

An overall strength training program, working both the upper and lower body, is important for football players at all levels. Use lighter weights and complete many repetitions. This approximates what you will do during the game better than trying to lift a heavy weight once.

Football is a "stop-and-go" sport, with intense activity followed by short rest periods. Maintain your nutrition with the Healthy Plate, and during the season, use the Training Plate. If you play in a weekly touch football game or flag football league, you need to keep your nutrition intake up during the days you do strength training. Carbohydrates are your fuel; protein builds and repairs muscles; and good fats are filling and satisfying.

If you need to snack, think whole fruit, such as apples and bananas with three-quarters cup of low-fat cottage cheese or yogurt; a handful of nuts and raisins; two tablespoons of nut butter on a piece of whole-grain toast; lettuce roll-ups with turkey, avocado, and mustard; or a protein shake or smoothie made with plain Greek yogurt, fruit, and one to two tablespoons of almond butter.

Football players need to take dehydration seriously, especially during pre-season and the very beginning of the season when temperatures are high and you are wearing all that equipment. Dehydration can cause overheating, reduced reaction time, cramps, muscle tears, and decreased strength and endurance. Hydration isn't just for practice and games; staying hydrated all day is very important. During practice or a game, aim for up to twenty ounces of fluid per hour, and drink something every fifteen to twenty minutes. For any practice or game lasting more than an hour, consider added electrolytes in the form of a sports drink, or something as simple as a banana or a handful of pretzels, especially if you sweat heavily.

Golf

A golfer's score is ultimately determined by athletic talent, by the amount of time devoted to practicing and playing, and physical fitness level. Unfortunately, most golfers overlook the fitness component and try to get by on natural talent and regular play. However, the more rounds you play without working on your conditioning, the greater are your chances of injury.

Strength is just as important in golf as accuracy. If you use your large trunk muscles when hitting the ball, you can generate much more power than you can with the smaller muscles of the arms and shoulders. Leg and back strength are equally important. To generate power as you pull the club through the swing, you need strong shoulders, and the forearms and wrists are particularly important in golf because they are used to give the ball added impetus.

Golfers can expect to be out on the course for four to five hours in an eighteen-hole round, so it's important to eat a nutritious meal beforehand to maintain blood sugar and energy levels to prevent fatigue throughout the round. Each golfer is different, but I suggest you eat a pre-round meal around three to four hours ahead, again, with an "Elvis bagel" or the equivalent.

Carry a small, healthy snack in your golf bag to top off energy levels and maintain concentration. Good snacks to have in your golf bag include fresh fruit, such as a banana; simple sandwiches (peanut butter and jelly, ham and cheese); dried fruit and mixed nuts; or salted pretzels.

On a hot summer day, dehydration can lead to fatigue, reduced skill performance, and impaired ability to focus and concentrate for longer periods. As golf is largely a game of skill and requires a high level of sustained concentration over several hours, make sure to drink adequate amounts of fluid to maintain good hydration levels while you play. Some golfers seem to benefit from a small amount of caffeine at the turn toward the back nine to aid skill and concentration. The ideal dose should be as small as possible to avoid side effects.

Hockey and Lacrosse

Hockey and lacrosse are sports that depend on leg strength and endurance, as well as strong wrists to generate power for most shots. Bigger, stronger players are better equipped to withstand the body contact these sports demand. Both upper-body and lower-body weight training is essential. Running long distances slowly can build aerobic conditioning and stamina. Intersperse these distances with intervals of sprints to improve speed.

The simple message for hockey and lacrosse players is get in your carbohydrates and protein and make sure you stay hydrated. Game-day nutrition is not just about pre-game, during game, and post-game strategies; you have to look at the big picture of what you are eating seven days a week. That's where the Healthy Plate and the Training Plate come in. This will prepare your body to train and also withstand the wear and tear of a long season and ensure that you have enough energy to put out your maximum effort every game.

In particular, I recommend the following foods for training for hockey and lacrosse players:

Fast-acting carbohydrates, best used in moderation during and after an event, include:

- Fruit juices
- Raisins

- Baked potatoes
- Watermelon
- Ripe bananas
- White rice
- Mashed potatoes
- Refined carbohydrate foods
- Quick oats
- Dried fruit

Prior to events and for weight management:

- Oranges
- Cereals
- Legumes
- Pasta
- Whole-grain breads

Slow-acting carbohydrates, best for maintaining blood sugar and weight management, include:

- Cherries
- Apples
- Leafy green vegetables
- Lentils
- Yogurt
- Steel-cut oatmeal

Running

Leg strength, obviously, is essential to runners. The exterior muscles in the leg drive your forward stride. The calves, hamstrings, quadriceps, buttocks, and lower-back muscles also need to be strengthened to improve your performance.

Distance running improves your stamina and conditioning. If you are interested in competitive running, even "fun runs," you need to do interval training, too, to increase your speed. Interval training is running for short bursts followed by a slow run. Take one or two days a week to do mostly interval training.

If you typically go for a run in the morning, what you eat beforehand is important; the morning meal before a running event is especially crucial. When I became founding medical director of the Rock 'n' Roll Marathon series, I came up with the concept of the "Elvis bagel." Ideally, if you eat something similar within two hours of running, you will feel better because you will be fully loaded with fuel.

The Healthy Plate will provide the rest of what you need in the form of stored glycogen for long-distance running (10K or more). For short distances (less than 10K), increase your fast-acting carbohydrates within one hour of the workout or race. Also, if you plan to do interval training, give yourself a little more fast-acting carbohydrates. To prepare for a future event, use the Training Plate.

Soccer

Soccer is a running game played on a huge field with practically no time allowed for rest. Cardiovascular conditioning is of the utmost importance. Soccer players are never out of the action for long. You may be able to rest momentarily when the play is across the field, but you are quickly on the go again. You need to work on your endurance, as well as agility and speed.

As part of your training, practice running both long distances and sprints. Or you can incorporate both into one workout. Jog for a quarter-mile and then sprint for fifty yards. Repeat to the point of muscle exhaustion. Work on your distance before you begin sprint work. This will give you a good aerobic base for sprinting.

Concentrate on strength-training workouts on the lower body. Exercises that strengthen the neck muscles can help with your headers.

Eating properly and hydrating adequately will ensure your stamina does not decrease quickly, which will slow you down, and allow you to deal with the physical and mental demands of soccer. The goal prior to a game is to maximize carbohydrate stores in the muscles and to top off blood sugar stores. Studies have shown that consuming fast-acting carbohydrate foods within an hour of exercise can actually lower blood sugar. Your body produces an "overshoot" of insulin and, in turn, causes low blood sugar. Before a match, soccer players should eat slow-acting carbohydrate foods to allow for a relatively slow release of sugar into the blood and avoid the insulin surge. Ideally, you should eat at least three hours prior to kickoff, especially if nerves are a factor, which can impair digestion.

Soccer players can lose between two to three liters of sweat during a game, particularly in hot and humid conditions. It's imperative that you drink plenty of fluids, preferably water, beforehand, and take in more fluid during breaks in the action and at half time.

Swimming

Swimming is probably the most nearly perfect form of exercise, especially at the recreational level. It's a non-weight-bearing exercise and poses no stress on the bones and joints, it strengthens the upper and lower body, it's easy to reach the training range and maintain it, it's effective to control weight, and it's a form of meditation.

Swimmers rely on power, speed, and endurance, not only in competition but in practice. Swimming works all of the body parts, so you need a total-body conditioning program. Make sure shoulder-strengthening and leg-strengthening exercises are part of your regular workout routine. A few minutes of stretching before and after swimming will make your stroke smoother and more efficient and will help relieve muscle soreness.

My sport has always been swimming. I was a lifeguard in day camp and a swim instructor, and I have always loved swimming. One question I get often from swimmers is, "Can I lose weight?" In a nutshell, the answer is "Yes." As long as you continue to kick and pull with your arms and limit your glide, you will raise your heart rate and burn calories. Concentrate on constantly moving in the water, and you can lose weight—if you also use the Healthy Plate to eat healthily.

You can tweak the carbohydrates on the Healthy Plate, depending on the distances you swim. For example, if you plan to do sprints of 25 to 50 meters that day, say, as part of interval training, think about adding a little more fast-acting carbohydrates into your pre-swim meal. If you are swimming distances of 200 to 400 meters slowly, you don't need to have as many fast-acting carbohydrates. Stick with the proportions of slow-acting and fast-acting carbohydrates in the Healthy Plate.

Tennis

The best way to improve your tennis game is not simply to play more tennis. You need a total-body strengthening program to help you hit the ball harder, move faster, and beat the players who are now beating you. In tennis, muscle strengthening has to be accompanied by muscle stamina. That is built by using light weights and doing many repetitions.

Running is an integral part of tennis. Wind sprints are particularly good for training. Also work on agility to improve your ability to change direction quickly.

I have found many weekend tennis players never eat properly before playing. Some don't eat at all if they have an early morning match. If you just drink a cup of coffee and go out and play, you are not fueling your body enough to play at your best. Between one and two hours beforehand, have an "Elvis bagel" or the equivalent. Within one hour of playing, add in more fast-acting carbohydrates, but not too much to get a sugar rush. I recommend tennis players eat fruit, for example, oranges, apples, tangerines, peaches, or plums. These fast-acting carbohydrates will keep you strong even into a third set.

If you have an upcoming tennis tournament, use the Training Plate the week before. Tennis is not really an endurance sport because the actions require fast movement. Bring some fruit with you to eat during the match, for example, seedless grapes. Seedless grapes are convenient, and you get a little more sugar than bananas. If you have been eating from the Training Plate, with a variety of leafy green vegetables and fruits, you have enough potassium and don't need any extra potassium from a banana. When you break between sets, have a piece of fruit. Drink fluids during the breaks as well. Remember to also check that you are hydrated well. In the heat of the match, you may forget the basics.

Triathlon

Anyone who enjoys fitness and takes the time to train can complete a triathlon, which consists of three events—swimming, cycling, and running, one after the other in succession. The triathlon brings into play virtually every part of the body, which makes it probably the most complete sporting event. As a general conditioning sport, the triathlon is much better than any of its three separate components. Each of the three sports requires good aerobic training, but there is little crossover from the lower to the upper body in aerobic training. Triathletes train both the lower body and the upper body aerobically. They also need a total-body strength training program.

Cramping due to muscle fatigue is a common problem for triathletes. Drink lots of liquids and eat from the Training Plate the week before a race to avoid this problem. If you know you are prone to muscle cramping, eat more potassium-rich foods, such as bananas, oranges, and tomatoes, a few days before an event to help prevent your muscles from suddenly cramping.

Some triathletes suffer from anemia due to iron deficiency or have digestive tract problems because they tamper with their diets to produce the maximum amount of energy. Others become vegetarians without understanding the potential dangers of dietary restrictions. Avoiding fish and chicken can rob your body of valuable protein, calcium, and iron. (See Chapter 7 for more on vegetarianism.) Triathletes need a balanced diet that is high in carbohydrates, rich in iron, and has large amounts of protein and calcium. Does this sound familiar? It should, because that's the Training Plate!

Volleyball

Power, which is a combination of strength and speed, is critical in volleyball. With all the fast, explosive movements that characterize the game, it may not seem as if volleyball players need to be strong, but overall body strength is quite important. You must not only develop your legs to help you jump higher, but you need to work your upper body as well to strengthen the back and shoulders. Train with weights to maintain strength and power.

I recommend eating one hour before a volleyball practice or match, again with an "Elvis bagel" or the equivalent. In a volleyball tournament format, you will play several games throughout one day. Take along easy-to-digest snacks, such as fresh fruit, cereal bars, or homemade gorp, to top off muscle glycogen stores for fuel. If you play several games in close succession, have a snack within thirty to sixty minutes of the end of each game to maintain optimal performance right through to the end of the tournament.

Good hydration is essential for sustained performance in volleyball. Drink frequently before and after games, and use the urine test to make sure you are properly hydrated. If you're playing beach volleyball in the hot sun, make sure to drink liquids before and after each game. During play, stop every fifteen minutes to have something to drink.

To sum up, understand that food is your fuel to participate in whatever sport you are doing. You know you need fuel. Using the Healthy Plate should give you everything you need as a base level. Using the Training Plate can give you that extra edge as you train for a long training day or for an event.

Make sure to eat something about two hours before a game with the equivalent of an "Elvis bagel." My special tweak during halftime or in between periods is to eat some fruit to hold off using up your glycogen stores. We have become familiar with soccer moms bringing orange slices for their kids to eat during halftime or after games. Sports scientists have now shown that having fructose on board makes the body's metabolism work better, and, therefore, Mom knew best—oranges are better than sports drinks for quick energy.

Drink plenty of fluids to ward off dehydration. Use the urine color test to know whether you are hydrated or not, and adjust your fluid intake accordingly.

PART THREE

Fueling Plates for Everyone

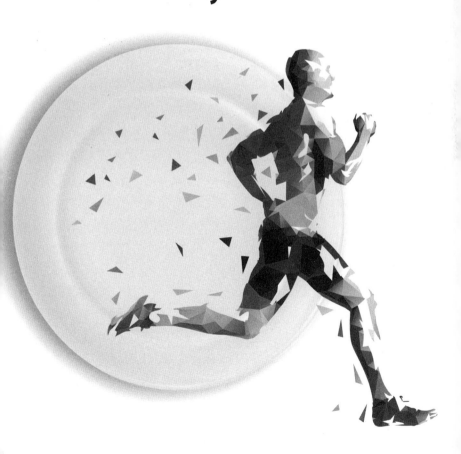

CHAPTER THIRTEEN

Fueling Plates for Women

Women often need slightly different eating patterns for more energy than men, and they may need to pay special attention in certain situations to perform at their best.

If a man and woman did the exact same amount of exercise and they were the exact same weight and had the exact same percentage of body fat, they would burn the same exact number of calories. But, in general, men tend to be larger, weigh more, and burn more calories during exercise. Men tend to have a higher percentage of muscles and as a result have a higher amount of lean body weight. It takes more calories to maintain muscle than fat, and men tend to eat more to maintain muscles. Again, in general, women tend to need fewer calories than men.

Because of the differences in body composition and food intake, women may cut down on the height of the basic food groups on their Fueling Plates. Women tend to have a higher percentage of body fat and therefore have higher amounts of energy stores. They, therefore, can be a little more choosy in what they eat and not eat as much since they have stored energy already on board.

Women tend to get iron deficiency once they reach childbearing age. During menstruation, women lose blood, and iron is found in the blood. An adult pregnant woman requires eighteen milligrams of iron daily, while an adult man of the same age requires only eight milligrams of iron daily. All vegetarian women may find it harder to get adequate amounts of iron from food they eat and therefore may need supplements. The most iron is found in a diet that is rich in meat, fish, and poultry. I suggest that vegetarian women supplement their iron intake with one iron pill a day; the exact dosage of iron should be discussed with your primary care physician, based on the results of blood tests.

Salad for Lunch

Debbie, a thirty-four-year-old advertising executive, wanted to beat her best time of five hours, twelve minutes at the New York City Marathon. We went over the Healthy Plate and the Training Plate and focused on her fueling. "I'm a salad person. How am I going to do these plates at lunch?" she asked. I suggested Debbie simply add in some protein to her salads. "But I just want to eat salad," said Debbie. I suggested she try the Healthy Plate and Training Plate and see how it feels in training.

"I continued to eat salads, with extra protein, for lunch for the month before the race. I didn't gain any weight, and I felt stronger when I was running. I finished the marathon in four hours and thirty-three minutes. I attribute most of the difference in my time to my improved eating patterns," said Debbie.

If you usually have a salad for lunch, there's no reason why you can't make that part of your Healthy Plate. Some of my patients who eat salads tend to emphasize they do so to eat less food. When

I explain the Healthy Plate to them, and its variety of nutrients, they no longer just load up on vegetables. And when they do, they feel the difference.

You can easily make a salad your Healthy Plate at lunch. Just make sure you have some protein, for example, roasted turkey, chicken, or shrimp, not just lettuce (a slow-acting carbohydrate), as well as some fast-acting carbohydrates (perhaps some fruit), and healthy fat (often found in the dressing). Before you put the salad in a bowl, put all the food you plan to eat on a plate, and then divvy it up into the four sections of the Healthy Plate to see how much you plan to eat. If you have extra food, put it aside and save it for another time.

If you are worried about gaining weight because you are eating more by using the Healthy Plate, eating more lettuce will allow you to eat more food and not gain weight. The lettuce will increase your bulk, but not your weight. The important trick is to add in protein. This helps repair and strength muscles and provides a backup source of energy.

Folate, an Important Vitamin

One of the most important nutrients for women is folate, or folic acid. Folate is a B vitamin that's important for cell growth and metabolism. Your body needs folate to make red and white blood cells in the bone marrow, convert carbohydrates into energy, and produce DNA and RNA. Adequate folate intake is extremely important during periods of rapid growth, such as pregnancy, infancy, and adolescence.

Folic acid is particularly important for pregnant women to protect unborn babies against birth defects. You can get enough folic acid from eating certain foods, including green leafy vegetables, oranges, beans, spinach, and nuts, or from foods fortified with vitamins, such as breads, pastas, and cereals. You can also get folic acid in the form of a vitamin supplement. Look for 400 micrograms of folic acid, which is 100 percent of the daily value of folic acid. Women of childbearing age need 400 to 800 micrograms per day.

The federal Office of Women's Health in the Department of Health and Human Services states that certain groups of women do not get enough folic acid each day from food. Nearly one in three African American women do not get enough folic acid each day. Spanish-speaking Mexican American women often do not get enough, but interestingly Mexican American women who speak English usually get enough folic acid.

You can develop folic acid deficiency anemia from not getting enough folic acid in your diet. This can be corrected by eating well or taking a folate supplement. Some women complain because this is usually a big pill, but as mentioned above, there are plenty of foods and enriched foods that can provide you with enough folate. You just need to be conscious of incorporating these foods into your Healthy Plate.

This is yet another reason to make sure to eat a variety of foods to get a full complement of nutrients. Don't hone in on one food every day and every meal in exclusion of other foods. For example, oranges provide vitamin C and carbohydrates, but no protein. Grilled chicken gives you iron and protein, but no vitamin C or carbohydrates. This is just to show you that variety really is the key to eating healthily, in addition to food color, with your Healthy Plate.

Women's Health Issues

Federal guidelines list no differences in the nutritional needs of boys and girls until they reach puberty. Since women are bearers of children, this tends to drive their nutritional needs to be specific and slightly different than men and, therefore, their food choices need to be more well-thought-out. For example, pregnant women have to guard against eating too much sugar or fast-acting carbohydrate foods or they risk gestational diabetes.

One of the most important issues for women who train regularly is feeling bloated, which can be due to the hormonal changes associated with their period or menopause. I recommend women eat more asparagus, which has diuretic properties, to reduce bloating. Some women who are inveterate exercisers have trouble getting pregnant. If you play tennis each weekend day and several other times a week, you may need to cut down on your amount of exercise to maintain enough body fat to menstruate regularly. I recommend these women eat a slightly higher fat intake, such as the After-a-Long-Workout Plate.

Senior women exercisers need to move to keep their bones strong. I also recommend foods with calcium and vitamin D, such as low-fat milk, to counteract bone loss. Have your bone density checked at your annual physical for signs of osteopenia (bone loss) or osteoporosis (bone wasting), and take calcium supplements, if indicated.

Female Athlete Triad

Some women who train intensely and maintain a rigid diet may actually be hurting their athletic pursuits and their health. These women are at risk for a problem known as *female athlete triad*. Female athlete triad is a combination of three conditions: disordered eating, amenorrhea (absence of three to twelve consecutive menstrual periods), and osteoporosis. A female athlete can have one, two, or all three parts of the triad.

#1: Disordered Eating

Many female athletes try to lose weight as a way to improve their performance. This leads some to disordered eating from not eating enough calories to keep up with energy demands, avoiding certain types of "bad" food (such as high-fat food), and serious eating disorders, such as anorexia nervosa or bulimia nervosa.

Anorexia is a psychological disorder in which a person loses her appetite and eats very little food. Bulimia nervosa is an emotional disorder involving a distorted body image and an obsessive desire to lose weight, which leads to bouts of extreme overeating followed by depression and self-induced vomiting, purging, or fasting.

Coaches can be part of this problem. Up to two-thirds of coaches do not know how to recognize the female athlete triad. This is an important statistic because the symptoms of the triad can be subtle. I look for any signs of abnormal eating, such as whether a young female athlete tends to eat in private so no one sees how little she is eating, or scars on her knuckles caused by stomach acid when she purges and vomits, which occurs in bulimics. I ask her and her family about how much and when she is eating, and whether she is taking in enough food.

I have had cross-country runners and gymnasts tell me their coaches said they needed to eat less to get their weight down so that they could perform better. In most cases, this is not necessarily true. These young female athletes will not necessary run faster or jump higher by losing a few pounds.

The problem is, socialization says thinner is better. Our society idolizes women pursuing to-the-bone thinness. Young women, including athletes, often starve themselves down to high-fashion figures. The pressures of athletic competition combined with the cultural emphasis on thinness increases the risks for athletes to develop disordered eating.

Many young female athletes with eating disorders go undiagnosed. Some of the signs and symptoms include dieting in spite of weight loss, a preoccupation with food and weight, frequent trips to the bathroom during and after meals, using laxatives, brittle hair or nails, dental cavities (bulimia wears away tooth enamel by frequent vomiting), sensitivity to cold, low heart rate and blood pressure, and heart irregularities and chest pain. If you see someone who has the signs and symptoms of an eating disorder, talk about it with her and encourage her to seek treatment. If need be, enlist a friend, family member, teacher, coach, or doctor to help the young athlete recognize it and get her the help she needs. Eating disorders can be deadly, and usually require treatment from a psychologist who specializes in them and also possibly a dietitian to recommend proper nutrition.

#2: Amenorrhea

Women who have missed at least three menstrual periods in a row have amenorrhea, as do girls who have not begun menstruating by age fifteen. A combination of intense exercise and not eating enough food can lead to decreases in the hormones that regulate the menstrual cycle. The end result is a delay in a young female athlete's first period or her periods may become irregular or stop. Older women athletes who become excessively thin can also experience menstrual irregularities or have no periods at all. Many women who began running in their mid-teens and have run long distances through their twenties have found that they are having trouble getting pregnant in their thirties.

Lack of body fat is one of the causes. The body's fat tissues store and convert hormones, including reproductive hormones. To allow the natural rise and fall of hormones during the menstrual cycle, a woman must maintain a certain amount of body fat content. Too much exercise, along with an excessively rigorous diet, may reduce a woman's body fat and cause her to have menstrual problems. Non-menstruating women athletes tend to consume less protein and take in fewer calories each day than menstruating athletes.

Young female athletes usually don't discuss their periods with a male coach. All coaches need to be aware of the issue of potential amenorrhea and talk about it with their young female athletes.

#3: Osteoporosis

Osteoporosis is a weakening of the bones due to the loss of bone density and improper bone formation. Low estrogen levels, common in young female athletes, and poor nutrition, especially low calcium intake, can lead to osteoporosis. Not getting enough calcium as a young woman can have a lasting effect on how strong a woman's bones are later in life.

In addition, osteoporosis can affect a female athlete's career because it may lead to stress fractures and other injuries. As a sports medicine physician, when I see a young female athlete who has had two stress fractures within one year, I look for the female athlete triad. These women often think that the stress fracture is from working out too hard. But they may not have osteoporosis yet. It may be an abnormal eating pattern has softened their bones enough to lead to stress fractures. Eating from the Healthy Plate often builds up their bones to avoid future stress fractures.

Pregnancy Physiology 101

The physiological changes a woman's body goes through during pregnancy are very similar to those produced by strenuous exercise. Briefly, cardiac output increases by 30 percent to 50 percent over the nonpregnant resting state. Medical people divide the nine months of pregnancy into three trimesters, each three months long. The greatest cardiac output increase occurs during the first trimester when uterine blood flow is only slightly increased and before the placental vascular flow has begun. A maximal maternal blood volume is seen in the third trimester, giving the woman the ability to maximize cardiac output while working less.

While pregnant, your breathing rate during exercise also increases, especially in the third trimester. Because there is an increase in total body mass, additional oxygen is needed to perform any given activity.

Other normal physiological changes occur in your blood cells, including a reduction of hematocrit and a slight increase in hemoglobin concentration. There are endocrine-based changes of carbohydrate and steroid metabolism. Curvature of the lumbar spine and relaxation of the cartilages of the symphysis pubis are also seen and are to be expected.

In general, exercise brings about similar physiologic alterations during pregnancy. Changes for the cardiovascular and respiratory systems are most pronounced and less marked for the musculoskel-etal and endocrine systems. If pregnancy and exercise are combined, there is a double physiologic impact. This very fact has led doctors, rightfully so, to recommend that if a prospective mother has not been involved in a vigorous exercise program prior to pregnancy, she should not be encouraged to begin one during her pregnancy.

Practical Recommendations

If you currently engage in regular exercise, you should not be discouraged from continuing. We now know, with our emphasis on physical fitness, that exercise is good not only for the general health of the nonpregnant female, but also for the pregnant woman. Exercise helps assure an easier birth (in most cases) and a healthy fetus.

Let's discuss practical and unique recommendations during each trimester:

First trimester. Hot baths, whirlpools, and saunas are to be avoided, as high temperatures have been linked to birth defects. This is not the time to begin an exercise program, but if you exercise, do not change your routine. Summer exercise should be conducted in the cool morning hours, when there is light for outdoor activities, but the temperature has not peaked; for example, running after sunset when the temperature is cooler carries with it the increased risk of injury due to darkness. Do not over-exert and run a marathon for a personal best. The greatest cause of heat stroke (and raised body temperature during running) is pushing too far; take it easy and hydrate appropriately. Prospective mothers should avoid medications, drugs, and tobacco and alcohol use. Medications should only be taken if deemed necessary and prescribed by a physician who knows you are pregnant.

Second trimester. All the same recommendations continue as in the first trimester. In the second trimester, the mother should start strengthening muscles used in labor and afterward, such as Kegel exercises. Your diet should be augmented with iron and calcium supplementation as the developing fetus begins to demand these elements in increasing amounts. A good physical examination by an obstetrician-gynecologist is critical to determine the competency of the cervix. This is the mouth of the uterus and helps hold the baby inside. If this is deemed "weak," it is the most common contraindication for vigorous exercise from now until the baby is born. Make sure that after your exam, you get cleared to exercise by your practitioner.

Third trimester. Research has shown that continued exercising during the third trimester is not harmful to the developing child. However, you should avoid exercises that may compromise fetal blood flow, particularly venous return, for example, standing in place for long periods of time and lifting heavy weights. Ideal exercises in addition to running that may be conducted include yoga, walking, and swimming (until near term but certainly not after rupture of the membranes).

A pregnant runner's diet shouldn't look too different from a nonpregnant runner's diet. Fill up your Healthy Plate with the same foods you have been eating. The same sources of fuel for energy you use for training will work while you are pregnant, too.

Leafy green vegetables should be one of the mainstays of your diet during pregnancy. Spinach and kale are high in folic acid, iron, fiber, and even fluids. Smoothies and soups are other good ways to stay hydrated, and add in healthy slow-acting carbohydrates in the form of vegetables, and fast-acting carbohydrates found in fruits. Focus on quality proteins, such as soy, eggs, lean meats, fish, poultry, and beans and grains.

A healthy pregnancy means weight gain, even while exercising. Plan on gaining twenty to thirty pounds, including the baby him- or herself. Pregnancy boosts your energy needs by about 300 calories a day, sometimes more during the end of the third trimester. If you exercise, you need to raise the height of the foods on your Healthy Plate to offset the calories burned during exercise so that you continue to put on needed weight and help your baby grow properly. For example, add in 200 to 300 calories for each half-hour of moderate activity, such as walking or swimming. Regular exercise increases your need for slow-acting carbohydrates, so add a little more slow-acting carbohydrates to your Healthy Plate. Also, pregnant women need even more fluids than they normally do. Replace any extra fluids you lose through sweat during exercise and check your urine color to make sure you are properly hydrated.

Postpartum. So now the baby has been born, what next? Depending on the type of delivery and the "normality" of delivery events, an exercise program should be resumed as shortly after delivery as is felt comfortable by both the mother and attending physician or nurse-midwife. Even while still in the hospital, you can begin to restore muscular tone to your abdomen and pelvis. This helps prevent urinary incontinence, uterine prolapse, and enhances a return to normal sexual activity. Exercise also promotes blood flow, avoiding such complications as varicose veins, leg cramps, edema, and blood clot formation. Improved circulation promotes healing of traumatized pelvic tissues and strengthens uterine and pelvic ligaments and tendons. I recommend continued Kegel exercises to strengthen the pelvic floor.

As an added benefit, exercise in the postpartum period has been shown to decrease the incidence of postpartum depression. We all know how we feel if we don't exercise, so get those endorphins kicking in.

The major exercises to avoid postpartum are those that employ a knee-to-chest position. Complications, both neurological and vascular, have been reported with these positions, so stay away from them during this initial period until you are cleared by your physician.

Return to your Healthy Plate as soon as possible after giving birth to help you build up any strength you may have lost during your pregnancy. Once you get back into regularly training, use the Training Plate.

Menstrual Irregularities

Menstrual irregularities among extreme exercisers have long been recognized. Amenorrhea (absence of three to twelve consecutive menstrual periods) and oligomenorrhea (irregular, infrequent menstruation, such as six to nine menstrual periods per year, or cycle length less than ninety days, but greater than thirty-five days) have both been seen in exercising women in all sports. Up to half of all women runners may see this happen to their periods.

Increased exercise causes a decreased pulsatile release of a hormone from the hypothalamus (gonadotropin-releasing hormone or GnRH), which leads to decreased luteinizing hormone (LH) and follicle-stimulating hormone (FSH) from the pituitary gland, which control your menstrual cycle.

The risk factors associated with this include: increased exercise intensity, prepubertal training; delayed onset of initial period; low body weight or weight loss; low body fat or fat loss; never having carried a pregnancy to term; never used oral contraceptive pills; a diet deficient in protein and total calories; history of a disordered eating pattern, such as bulimia or anorexia; family history of amenorrhea and/or oligomenorrhea; and psychological stress. The more risk factors you have, the more likely you are to have an irregular or absent period.

The exact cause of the decreased GnRH is still under discussion among fertility experts. Causes thought to be involved include beta-endorphins and other hormones in the body that increase with exercise.

You need to have a thorough evaluation and treatment plan for menstrual dysfunction. If left unchecked and brushed off as a normal consequence of exercising, it can lead to osteoporosis, stress fractures, increased growth of the endometrium (leading to heavier, more painful periods later on), and soft-tissue injuries.

Your physician should evaluate your training schedule and any changes in it over the past six months or the time you are having menstrual irregularity. A full diet evaluation should be done, as well as a record of what drugs you are taking and whether you have had recent stress fractures or psychological stress.

Next up is the laboratory evaluation. Your doctor will probably order a urine pregnancy test (if indicated), and check your blood levels of thyroid stimulating hormone and prolactin; a progestin challenge test to indicate whether you have adequate amounts of circulating estrogen in your body; and FSH and LH blood levels if the progestin challenge test is negative. If your FSH and LH blood levels are high, this indicates ovarian failure and not a hormonal problem. If FSH and LH are low, you likely have athletic amenorrhea.

The treatment is simple. Although decreasing training and increasing weight usually solves the problem, I know few runners who go for this plan. Hormonal treatment to bring on periods every three months, or using oral contraceptives, are an alternative that some obstetrician-gynecologists feel comfortable prescribing. As a good first step, make sure your protein intake is good (use the Healthy Plate), along with adequate calcium (1500 milligrams daily). If stress is involved, a referral to a good psychologist sometimes will help.

The next chapter will go over the concerns of young athletes, both boys and girls.

CHAPTER FOURTEEN
Fueling Plate for Teens

Young teens, both boys and girls, going through growth spurts need to eat more. They must make sure to follow a healthy diet to raise their metabolism as they grow. Many adolescents also have what's known as the "Superman Syndrome"—they believe they can eat anything without harming themselves and say they know what to eat. Yet most adolescents don't know what they don't know about good nutrition. That's why the Healthy Plate and Training Plate are essential for young athletes to follow.

Sports Nutrition for Young Athletes

Jeff, a sixteen-year-old cross-country runner on his high school team, came to see me with his coach, Bruce. "Jeff has great form, and trains a lot, but he is not winning any meets," said Bruce. I asked Jeff what he normally eats for lunch, and he told me, "Chicken nuggets, Cheetos, and a large sports drink."

I set up Jeff with the Healthy Plate. He understood the concepts, and having his coach support him in using the Healthy Plate gave it even more credibility. "I started eating better with the Healthy Plate, and my times improved. The only thing different was my eating pattern," said Jeff. He became a top runner and was offered a scholarship to run at Syracuse University. "I never would have gotten to that level without changing my diet," said Jeff.

Nutrition is important for the performance of young athletes, as well as for optimal growth and development. They need the macronutrients of the Healthy Plate—slow-acting carbohydrates, fast-acting carbohydrates, protein, and fat—as well as micronutrients, such as vitamins and minerals, and fluids before, during, and after exercise. Using the Healthy Plate allows even adolescents to make sure they are eating properly.

Before puberty, young children have more energy than you ever thought possible. In order to do that, they have to eat to get the maximum amount of energy. Most young children eat intuitively to maximize their energy output.

As children go through puberty, the nutritional requirements are the same, but they need more food. In general, young male athletes need to eat more food than young female athletes because they expend more energy. A 65-pound girl who plays soccer for 60 minutes expends 270 calories. A 125-pound boy playing ice hockey for 60 minutes expends 936 calories. This tells you that they have different nutrient needs to maintain enough energy for their sports.

Basic nutrition is important for adolescents to grow, achieve good health, and to provide energy for their chosen sport. Good nutrition enhances athletic performance by decreasing fatigue and the risk of disease and injury. It enables young athletes to optimize training and recover faster. Balancing energy intake with energy expenditure is crucial to prevent an energy deficit or excess. Energy deficits can cause short stature, delayed puberty, menstrual dysfunction, loss of muscle mass, and increased susceptibility to fatigue, injury, or illness. Energy excess can result in becoming overweight or obese.

The key is to make sure that adolescents eat a balanced diet to get all the nutrients they need. The best way is to practice using the Fueling Plates. Have your adolescent athlete draw the outline of the Healthy Plate and imagine putting foods into it. After they do this a few times, they will get it. Encourage them to use the Healthy Plate during lunch at school and at dinner at home.

Micronutrients

Young athletes need many vitamins and minerals for good health but should pay particular attention to consuming proper amounts of calcium, vitamin D, and iron.

Calcium is important for bone health, to normalize enzyme activity, and for muscle contractions. Calcium is found in a variety of foods and beverages, including milk, yogurt, cheese, broccoli, spinach, and fortified grain products.

Vitamin D is necessary for bone health and also for the absorption and regulation of calcium. Young athletes living in northern latitudes or who train indoors, for example, hockey players and gymnasts, are more likely to be vitamin D deficient. Good sources of vitamin D in addition to sun exposure include fortified foods, such as milk. Many dairy products other than milk, such as yogurt, do not contain vitamin D.

Iron is important to deliver oxygen to body tissues. During adolescence, more iron is required to support growth as well as increases in blood volume and lean muscle mass. Iron depletion is common in young athletes because of diets that lack enough protein from meat, fish, and poultry, or increased iron losses in the urine, feces, sweat, or menstrual blood. Adolescent athletes, particularly female athletes, vegetarians, and distance runners, should be screened periodically to make sure they have proper iron levels in their blood. Iron-rich foods include eggs, leafy green vegetables, fortified whole grains, and lean meat.

Quality, Not Quantity

Susan brought her son Damon, age seventeen, to see me so I could tell him exactly what to eat for lacrosse. I had him write out the Healthy Plate and Training Plate on the paper of my exam table, and Damon practiced how he would put different foods onto the plates and how high each section should be.

Two weeks later they came in again for a checkup, and Damon said, "I felt bloated during games, and I threw up at half time." I asked him what he was drinking and he said, "I had a sports drink before and after each game." I suggested he drink only water and cut back on the amount of each section on the Healthy Plate and Training Plate. "I stopped the sports drinks and used both plates with less food, and felt great during games. I had more energy to last the whole game," said Damon.

Sometimes it's a matter of quality, not quantity, to get the right amounts of food to be healthy. The quality of the foods an adolescent puts on his or her Fueling Plate is more important than the quantity since most young athletes eat a lot. As mentioned above, micronutrients, including calcium, vitamin D, and iron, are particularly important if young athletes are still growing, which may continue into their early twenties.

I often have to teach active adolescents how to stay well hydrated so that their bodies function properly. Adolescent athletes also have greater water needs than do adult athletes. Adolescents often think drinking sports drinks is fine, but drinking too many sports drinks can cause bloating. I encourage them to look at the color of their urine to know whether they are hydrated. I explain why they need fluids and talk directly to them, not their parents. They usually get it right away.

Athletic performance can be affected by what, how much, and when a young athlete drinks. As we discussed in Chapter 2, fluids help to regulate body temperature and replace sweat losses during exercise. Environmental temperature and humidity can affect how much an adolescent athlete sweats and how much fluid intake is required. Hotter temperatures and higher humidity also affect how much they sweat, and more fluid may be needed to maintain hydration. Dehydration can decrease performance and put adolescent athletes at risk for heat exhaustion or heat stroke.

If an adolescent athlete is competing in an all-day event, say, a volleyball tournament, then the use of a sports drink may be warranted. Otherwise, if they are exercising less, water is fine to maintain hydration.

Skipping meals is a common phenomenon among adolescents. Because of their busy schedules during and after school, adolescents may grab junk foods and eat sparingly of quality foods, and then catch up on food intake during the late evening. Timing of food consumption is important to optimize performance. Meals should be eaten a minimum of three hours before exercise, and snacks should be eaten one to two hours before activity. Regular use of the Healthy Plate ensures the adolescent athlete is getting the right amounts of high-quality foods.

Fatigue

Fatigue is also a common problem among young athletes. Teens need sleep to help their bodies grow. They also need extra energy from food to help their bodies grow, and this comes from a good, healthy diet, like the one provided by following the Healthy Plate. They need even more energy during training, and that's where the Training Plate comes in.

Some teens lack sufficient iron in their bodies. Even though their iron deficiency may not be severe enough to produce anemia, it can slow their growth, deplete their energy supply, and lead to poor sports performance. Iron deficiency is usually associated with young female athletes, but young male athletes also lose iron during strenuous exercise.

In general, I don't recommend vitamin supplements for young athletes. Most of them eat enough, and as long as they eat a balanced diet, they do not need vitamin supplements. A balanced, varied diet through the Healthy Plate provides adequate calories and nutrition to meet the needs of most adolescent athletes.

I recommend that adolescent athletes carry snacks with them to school to supplement their lunch. For example, a bag of dried fruits and nuts, a peanut butter and jelly sandwich on whole-wheat bread, fruits, such as a few handfuls of grapes, or even whole-grain trail mix can help stave off fatigue and hunger pangs after school before sports practice starts and provide a quick pick-me-up right after practice.

Recovery foods are particularly important for adolescent athletes to consume within thirty minutes of exercise, and again within one to two hours of exercise, to help reload muscles with glycogen and allow for proper recovery. These foods should include protein and carbohydrates, for example, graham crackers with peanut butter and juice, yogurt with fruit, or fruit and cheese.

Body Image

Rebecca, a nineteen-year-old college cross-country runner, came in to see me specifically to talk about sports nutrition. "I want to increase the size of my body. Everyone says I look like a pencil," said Rebecca. "I can run more miles than anyone else on the team. I think I eat well to give me the energy I need."

I asked Rebecca to keep a food diary for one week. She wrote down what she ate, including the size and amount of food, for example, one small orange for snack right after practice. When she came back, we discussed the Fueling Plates, and she practiced drawing some. We talked about how high to pile up food on the plates.

"It turned out I was barely eating enough to maintain my energy level, but not enough to gain weight. I used the Fueling Plates during the week and just before and after meets, and I gained five pounds in a month. I felt stronger during meets and much better about my body image," said Rebecca.

There has always been more pressure on young women to look a particular way. Young women of all ages do the "fat talk." They get together and talk about each other's bodies, saying things like, "I'm fat. My thighs are too big." This leads to body image problems. When young female athletes talk negatively about their bodies over and over again, they become dissatisfied with their bodies. This type of thinking often leads to other thoughts like, "I need to lose weight." And this can lead a young athlete to develop an eating disorder.

A recent survey conducted by ESPN of Division I National Collegiate Athletic Association athletes found that nearly one-third of female athletes reported that they lie about their weight sometimes, 20 percent reported being called "fat" by at least one coach, and more than two-thirds said they feel pressured to look "pretty" even when they are competing. These attitudes place them at risk for anorexia nervosa. Most athletes with eating disorders are female, but male athletes are also at risk, especially those competing in sports that tend to place an emphasis on diet, appearance, size, and weight requirements, such as running, wrestling, and crew.

One way I detect body image problems, and often associated eating disorders, is to put a young female athlete on a scale so that she can see her own weight. I can often tell poor body image is an issue just by her reaction—"That's way too high!" When I do make the diagnosis of eating disorders, I refer to a psychologist who specializes in treating eating disorders.

Part of the treatment of poor body image goes back to fuel. Food is like the gas in your tank. Put in "high test" food and your body engine will respond by performing at top efficiency. The Healthy Plate for regular meals and the Training Plate during peak exercise times provide that type of fuel for young athletes.

The last chapter discusses the importance of Fueling Plates for particular medical conditions—heart disease, diabetes, and kidney disease.

CHAPTER FIFTEEN

Fueling Plates for Heart Disease, Diabetes, and Kidney Disease

*T**his chapter includes advice* for those with specific medical conditions that require dietary attention. Heart disease patients need to follow a heart-healthy diet—that's what the Healthy Plate provides—to limit their fat and cholesterol intake and to watch how much salt they eat.

Diabetics need to know how much sugar they can eat or drink throughout the day. We will go over the potential dangers of sports drinks, which may cause a diabetes patient to go into a diabetic coma because of a too-high-sugar content; the use of a portable blood-sugar monitor now available to know how much sugar is in your blood; and the importance of continuing to exercise with diabetes and also eating from the Healthy Plate.

Another medical condition that requires a special diet includes those with kidney problems, who need less protein and other micro-nutrients in their diets.

Heart Disease Risk Factors

Several health conditions, your lifestyle, your age, and family history can increase your risk for heart disease, which are called risk factors. About half of all Americans (47 percent) have at least one of the three key risk factors for heart disease: high cholesterol, high blood pressure, and cigarette smoking. You can't control some of the risk factors for heart disease, but you can take steps to lower your risk by changing the factors you can control.

For adults, risk factors for heart disease include being overweight or obese; an unhealthy diet (using Fueling Plates provides you with a healthy diet); cigarette smoking; a sedentary lifestyle; age and gender—if you are over age forty-five years for men and over age fifty years for women; high blood pressure of 140/90 mm mercury or higher; family history of heart disease; and any preexisting heart disease, diabetes, or prediabetes. You have less of a risk of heart disease if your "good" high-density lipoprotein (HDL) cholesterol level is higher than 60 mg/dL.

Some major risk factors you cannot change include your age, gender, and heredity. But the majority of heart disease risk factors are modifiable, including cigarette smoking, cholesterol level, blood pressure level, blood sugar level, weight, physical activity level, and diet.

So how do you know which risk factors you have? Your doctor may conduct or request screening tests during regular visits. It's unlikely you will have ideal risk levels on all screening tests, however, if you do have test results that are less than ideal, it doesn't mean you're destined to develop a serious heart condition. What it means is you are in a position to begin changing your health in a positive way.

Your body weight and blood pressure are usually taken at every routine medical exam beginning at age twenty. The frequency of follow-up will depend on your level of heart disease risk. A lipid profile to measure your total, HDL cholesterol, and "bad" low-density lipoprotein (LDL) cholesterol levels is generally done every four to six years for normal-risk adults. This may be done more often if you have elevated risk factors for heart disease and stroke. You may have your waist circumference measured to help evaluate your risk if your body mass index is greater than or equal to 25 kg/m², which is considered to be overweight. Your doctor should ask about smoking, your physical activity level, and diet at every regular visit.

Blood sugar tests are done at least every three years. The American Diabetes Association recommends testing for prediabetes and your risk for future diabetes beginning at age forty-five. If tests are normal, it is reasonable to repeat testing at a minimum of three-year intervals.

The American Academy of Pediatrics recommends that children have their cholesterol checked between age nine and eleven, and adolescents should have it checked again from ages seventeen and twenty-one. This is to pick up any potential bad eating habits or hereditary disorders that may increase the child's risk of high cholesterol levels later in life.

Running with Heart Disease

"I had a heart attack ten years ago and my cardiologist doesn't like the idea of me running," says Eugene, a sixty-seven-year-old salesman. *"All of my cholesterol levels and stress tests are fine, but I have three clogged arteries, one at 40 percent and two at 30 percent. I don't eat a*

lot of fried foods and drink a glass of red wine every night to help raise my HDL cholesterol. I want to keep running!"

As there is no proven benefit to marathon running in preventing heart attacks, the general advice by exercise-savvy cardiologists is that you can exercise, but with caution, always paying attention to your body, and seeking help should there be any form of chest discomfort (not necessarily pain) that occurs with effort. The long duration of a marathon (four hours or more for the average older runner) may be too much of a stress on obstructed arteries. If despite this, you decide to run a marathon, you should definitely get a stress test first to make sure the effort of running a long race is not too dangerous.

You may have heard stories of top runners and other professional athletes having a heart attack or dying suddenly from heart disease. Champion marathon runner Alberto Salazar had a heart attack at age forty-eight. His having a heart attack and needing coronary artery stents for clogged arteries invites the questions: Should someone with coronary artery disease run? And is running really good for you or in any way protective against heart disease?

Another famous case is Jim Fixx, the runner and best-selling author. Even though he was a runner and died at age fifty-two, Fixx survived nine years longer than his father, who died of a heart attack at age forty-three. Apparently, Fixx's total cholesterol level was higher than 250 mg/dL and he deferred getting a stress test, even though cardiologist Kenneth Cooper, MD, who pioneered the benefits of doing aerobic exercise for maintaining and improving health, recommended he have one. An autopsy revealed blockage in Fixx's three main arteries of 95 percent, 85 percent, and 50 percent.

Sudden Cardiac Death

The tragedy of exercise-related death is fortunately a rare occurrence that may strike young, asymptomatic, and seemingly healthy athletes. Well-known examples besides Jim Fixx include the deaths of basketball players Hank Gathers and Reggie Lewis, and Minnesota Vikings offensive tackle Korey Stringer. Such incidents have increased the awareness of exercise-related death, raised questions about proper preparticipation screening for athletes, and prompted studies into the incidence and causes of exercise-related death.

Physicians define "sudden death" in young athletes (ages thirty-five and younger) as a nontraumatic, nonviolent, unexpected death due to cardiac causes within one hour of the onset of symptoms. One study estimated that the incidence of sudden cardiac death in unscreened men during exercise is one in 280,000 per year. In studies of the risk of death in marathons, it's been estimated that one death would occur in 50,000 to 88,000 marathon finishers. In a study I published with Dr. Steve Van Camp in 2004, we found that the risk in distances between 10K and half-marathon was significantly lower, only 3.1 deaths per million finishers.

The incidence of a sudden cardiac death is 56 times greater during exercise in sedentary men, yet only 5 times greater risk during exercise in active men. The risk of having a heart attack is 107 times greater with exercise in sedentary men and only 2.7 times greater with exercise in active men.

"Athlete's Heart"

Exercise causes normal blood flow and electrical changes seen on an electrocardiogram. During intense aerobic exercise, the oxygen consumption of muscle tissue increases, and the heart's output must rise to meet the demands. Over time, aerobic training results in beneficial changes in the heart, including increased left ventricular mass, decreased resting heart rate, increased ventricular stroke volume, and increased cardiac output, among other effects. This is called an "Athlete's Heart"—it is normal and nothing to worry about.

My sports cardiologist friends in New York City with an interest in exercise point out that the key points to understand are the duration and severity of exercise. Many older (age fifty and up) runners have undiagnosed coronary artery obstructions. Stress testing will only diagnose the severe lesions and not the mild and the moderate (less than 70 percent) obstructions. All plaques, severe or not, have the potential to rupture and cause a heart attack. The exact cause is not known, but it is believed that exercise can be a factor. This does not mean that exercise is not beneficial. It definitely is helpful but is not without some risk.

Runners are more at risk during the hour or so after they train. You are particularly at risk if you run marathons, as your time out on the road with an elevated heart rate increases. But the remainder of the day, all cardiologists agree, you are much less at risk than the general population, and running can actually extend and improve your life and lifestyle.

As a medical director of marathons, I hate to see a runner go down with a heart incident. If you run for an hour, play several hard sets of tennis, or play soccer all day, you are, in effect, doing your own stress test as if you were on a treadmill. The difference is you don't have someone safely monitoring your heart during this exercise period.

"Silent" Heart Attacks

There are two types of "silent" heart attacks, that is, without symptoms beforehand. If you have diabetes, you can have a heart attack and not even feel it. The other heart attack occurs with no angina, which is a type of chest pain caused by reduced blood flow to the heart and is a symptom of coronary artery disease. Angina symptoms—squeezing, pressure, heaviness, tightness, or pain in your chest—are often described as if an elephant is standing on your chest. There is no way to predict this type of a heart attack until the angina hits.

Heart Recommendations

I'm not a cardiologist; I am just presenting you with the basic facts. If you have further questions about heart disease and exercising, please talk about this with a cardiologist. My general recommendation includes don't be afraid of statins (cholesterol-lowering medications). Some athletes tend to think if they are exercising, they don't need to take statins. If you have a strong family history of heart disease, make sure you know your cholesterol numbers and do whatever it takes, including taking cholesterol-lowering medications, to get them under control (for more on cholesterol, see Chapter 3).

If you are running long distances at age forty or older, have a stress test and your cholesterol levels checked. You may have silent heart disease that can be exacerbated by an endurance event. Let your doctor know what type of exercise you plan to do and the length of the exercise. If you run a mile around the park twice a week, I would be less concerned than if you were training for a marathon, which puts more stress on the heart.

If you are in your thirties and plan to run a marathon for the first time and you have a family history of heart disease, say, your mother died of a heart attack at age sixty, I highly recommend you have a stress test before running the race. My point is that if you have a family history of heart disease, you may have heart disease regardless of how much you exercise.

If you have high cholesterol levels and think you could have a potential heart disease problem, you need to have blood tests and have regular checkups with a physician. Remember, even if you exercise regularly and eat a healthy diet with the Fueling Plates, a high proportion of heart disease is due to heredity, not lifestyle. You want to have as much background knowledge as you can about your heart health to stay healthy and live a long life. If you have heart disease risk factors, there's no good reason not to be proactive and do something to lower your risks.

Please remember that exercising is safe and healthy for the vast majority of people. Without exercise, you are likely to have a higher incidence of death, higher blood pressure, greater risk of heart disease and diabetes, and a lower overall quality of life.

So please don't stop exercising because you hear of an athlete dying suddenly. Most running events are proud that their medical staff involves a fleet of dedicated ambulances and paramedics stationed along the course, hundreds of medical volunteers at numerous stations throughout the course and start and finish lines, and a dedicated on-site communications and dispatch system. Indeed, if you were to have a heart attack during such an event, the safest place to be is in a hospital or on one of these race courses.

And bear in mind that in any population of 50,000 people — even ones just sitting around or doing yard work—a certain percentage will likely suffer heart attacks over that same several-hour time period. This is a point that seems lost on some who warn that exercise will "kill you."

What steps can you take today to support your heart health while exercising? I would recommend the following:

- Be sure to have an annual physical exam and tell the examiner exactly what you are training for, and how. If you are training for a race, indicate your training pace and your expected finishing time. All of that information may change the tests and how you are examined.

- If you develop new chest pain or more shortness of breath than usual during training or during an event, stop immediately and seek medical attention.

- Ask your doctor about taking a baby aspirin (81 mg) daily, or, at the very least, before any long event, if you have no contraindications. Anytime in the morning before your event is okay. Do not consume a nonsteroidal inflammatory drug, such as aspirin, during a run or walk of less than 10K or a short exercise bout.

- Only drink a sports drink during a 10K run or more, or the equivalent workout.

- Drink for thirst.

- I see no downside to limiting your caffeine intake on the day of a long event. High doses of caffeine have been implicated in setting off a fatal heart attack. Less than 200 mg (about two cups of coffee) seems to be the appropriate amount of caffeine beforehand.

- Consume salt (if you have no medical contraindication) during a 10K or longer race or longer exercise bout.

- Eat from the Fueling Plates to ensure you have a heart-
  healthy diet.

Fueling Plates for Heart Disease

Most general guidelines on a heart-healthy diet recommend
certain steps to prevent heart disease. These steps include:

- *Control your portion size.* The major point of using Fueling Plates is to not overload your plate, and if you do, to set
  aside any excess food to eat later. Then you will not eat until
  you feel stuffed, which can lead to eating more than you
  should and potentially gaining weight.
- *Eat more vegetables and fruits.* Vegetables and fruits contain substances that may help prevent heart disease. Eating
  more vegetables (slow-acting carbohydrates) and fruits
  (fast-acting carbohydrates) may help you cut back on higher
  calorie foods, such as meat, cheese, and snack foods.
- *Select whole grains.* Whole grains are good sources of fiber
  and other nutrients that play a role in regulating blood
  pressure and heart health. Simply substitute slow-acting
  carbohydrate whole-grain products (whole-grain bread,
  high-fiber cereal, brown rice) for fast-acting carbohydrates,
  such as refined-grain products (white bread, frozen waffles,
  egg noodles).
- *Limit unhealthy fats.* Limit how much saturated fat and
  trans fats you eat, and you will reduce your blood cholesterol and lower your risk of coronary artery disease. In general, stay away from fried foods since they contain lots of
  fat. For example, grilled chicken is better for you than fried

chicken. When you put protein onto your Fueling Plate, if it's fried, then some portion of the protein counts toward the fat portion of the Fueling Plate.

- *Choose low-fat protein sources.* Fish are rich in omega-3 fatty acids, which can lower levels of triglycerides, which have been implicated in heart disease. Other good choices include low-fat dairy products, eggs, legumes, soybeans, and lean ground beef.
- *Reduce the sodium in your food.* Eating too much sodium can contribute to high blood pressure, a risk factor for heart disease. Be wary of canned or processed foods, such as soups, baked goods, and frozen dinners, which often contain tons of salt. Use the Healthy Plate to cook your own fresh foods and soups to reduce the amount of salt you eat.

The idea of the Fueling Plates is not to think so hard about the foods you choose. If you organize the food on your plate as we have described, you will eat mostly fresh vegetables (slow-acting carbohydrates) and fruits (fast-acting carbohydrates), plus some healthy fats (such as avocado), and protein (as I mentioned above, grilled chicken or shrimp, and not as much fatty beef) to take into account a heart-healthy diet.

Diabetes

Stephanie, a thirty-five-year-old manager, had been competing in triathlons for ten years. "I was a competitive swimmer in high school and now enjoy triathlons. I was quite surprised when I found out at my last checkup that I have type 2 diabetes. Now I have to watch how much sugar I take in, and I take insulin daily. I can't imagine competing

in a triathlon and having to test my blood sugars during the race,"
said Stephanie.

Diabetes is usually classified into three categories. Type 1 and type 2 are the most common types worthy of discussion. Gestational diabetes only occurs among pregnant women.

Type 1 diabetes usually comes on early in life and is due to an autoimmune response causing a deficiency in insulin, which is needed to get sugar into cells. It can be diagnosed by a blood test showing the autoimmune process going on and by genetic markers. Type 1 diabetics need insulin every day.

Type 2 diabetes is basically a resistance to insulin that causes high sugar levels in the blood. These patients are often managed by a combination of dietary changes along with medications in pill form or insulin shots.

Gestational diabetes develops during pregnancy and also affects how your cells use sugar. In gestational diabetes, blood sugar levels usually return to normal soon after delivery, but if you have had gestational diabetes, you are at risk for type 2 diabetes.

There are many complications of long-term diabetes, including vision, kidney, and heart problems, along with foot ulcers, amputations, and neuropathy. With good blood sugar control, which includes using the Fueling Plates program, you can avoid serious complications.

Many professional athletes have been able to compete in their sport using good training procedures, practicing their insulin balance, and eating properly. Some of these famous professional athletes include football player Jay Cutler, basketball player Chris Dudley, baseball players Ron Santo and Jackie Robinson, and tennis players Arthur Ashe and Billie Jean King.

Huge numbers of endurance athletes, including marathoners and triathletes, have competed without checking their sugar during their race. I have heard of some doctors and some runners who want to test their blood sugar level during an endurance event. To me, this is ridiculous compulsivity. They are either not informed or just don't understand the nature of blood sugar control.

Training, as I have mentioned earlier in the book, is essentially practice for your chosen event. If you have diabetes, you need to check your blood sugar levels during training, as well as during eating and drinking, so you know what to expect on event day. You should be able to work up to five hours or more of exercise without having to stop to check your blood sugar level.

In order to best help you control your diabetes during sports, you need to find a sports medicine specialist or an endocrinologist to help you through your training and practice. You need to understand the importance of blood sugar control to prevent long-term complications, but you also need to know that you don't need to sacrifice performing in sports at a high level. Unfortunately, there is no one specific regimen to tell you how to do this. You are an experiment unto yourself. By practicing in training, I know you will not have to stop. And with the help of the Fueling Plates program, you will get your eating and drinking regimen down to a science and can continue to exercise with diabetes.

Blood Sugar Testing

The key to diabetes is to keep your blood sugar within normal limits. Everyone is different, so go over the individual levels with your doctor. The normal goal of blood sugar is between 150 and 250 mg/dl.

If you are diabetic, the best time to exercise is one to three hours after eating, when your blood sugar level is likely to be higher. If you use insulin, it's important to test your blood sugar before exercising. If the level before exercise is below 100 mg/dl, eat a piece of fruit or have a small snack to help you avoid hypoglycemia. During training, test again thirty minutes later to prove that your blood sugar level has stabilized. Then you will know what you need to eat before you compete in a long event.

Recheck your blood sugar level after a long workout or activity. If you take insulin, your risk of developing hypoglycemia may be highest six to twelve hours after exercising. Do not exercise if your blood sugar level is too high (over 250 mg/dl) because exercise may raise blood sugar levels even higher.

FreeStyle Libre

The FreeStyle Libre has revolutionized blood sugar monitoring. This system eliminates the hurdles of traditional glucose monitoring and requires no routine finger sticks or finger stick calibrations. The system measures glucose levels through a small sensor—the size of two stacked quarters—applied to the back of your upper arm. It provides real-time glucose readings for up to ten days, both day and night. The sensor can also read glucose levels through clothes, making testing discreet and very convenient if you are exercising.

It provides three critical pieces of data with each scan: a real-time glucose result; an eight-hour historical trend; and a directional trend arrow showing where glucose levels are headed. The touch-screen reader also holds up to ninety days of data, which allows you to track your glucose levels over time.

You can use the small reader that comes with the system or an app on your cell phone to get a snapshot if you are experiencing hypoglycemic trends (low glucose levels) or hyperglycemic trends (high glucose levels), which can aid in choosing the right diabetes management. Studies show those who use the FreeStyle Libre system spend less time in hypoglycemia as compared with those who managed their glucose with a traditional self-monitoring glucose system.

Fueling Plates for Diabetes

A healthy diet for diabetics includes eating the same variety of foods that contain the slow-acting carbohydrates, fast-acting carbohydrates, proteins, fats, vitamins and minerals, fiber, and water we discussed earlier. However, diabetics have to spend time each day to plan healthy meals. In general, think about including more non-starchy vegetables (beans and whole grains) into the Healthy Plate. Starchy vegetables (corn and potatoes) turn into more sugar in your body, and then you require more insulin.

Cut down on the amount of fast-acting carbohydrates, such as fruits. If you eat too many fruits, your blood sugar levels may yo-yo up and down. You want a more steady-state level.

Diabetics should also eat servings of low-fat or fat-free milk or milk substitutes, like almond milk, which have some sugar and protein in the milk. Concentrate on eating lower-fat protein, such as lean steak versus fatty short ribs. Be careful about how much sugar and direct fats (something you see directly as a fat, like butter) you are eating, in addition to hidden fats in sauces. Diabetics should cut down on the height of the fat part of the Healthy Plate.

Diabetes Recommendations

My general recommendations for diabetes patients who exercise regularly include:

- Make sure you test your blood sugar and, if prescribed, take your medication.
- Eat a low-sugar, low-fat diet by using the Healthy Plate.
- Cut down on your intake of sports drinks. Many sports drinks are filled with hidden sugar. I suggest you cut the amount of sports drinks in half, or dilute them with water.
- Do not stop exercising; in fact, exercise is highly recommended for diabetic patients. All types of exercise can help lower blood sugar levels.

Kidney Disease

Kidney disease means your kidneys are damaged and cannot filter blood the way they should. You are at greater risk for kidney disease if you have diabetes or high blood pressure. If you have kidney disease, you need to adjust your diet to accommodate for the decrease in the kidney's function to eliminate wastes.

The first thing to managing chronic kidney disease is to understand it better. What does it mean? In laymen's terms, chronic kidney disease is a gradual loss of kidney function. The kidneys play a key role in removing toxins from the body. Your kidneys filter wastes and excess fluids from your blood, which are then excreted in your urine. When chronic kidney disease reaches an advanced stage, dangerous levels of fluid, electrolytes, and wastes can build up in your body. The goal of treatment of chronic kidney disease is to slow down the decrease in function of the kidneys before they reach complete failure and you need dialysis or a kidney transplant.

A combination of dietary and lifestyle changes, including increased exercise, can help you accomplish this. The basic tenet of kidney disease diets is to restrict the amount of protein as well as sodium, potassium, and phosphorus in your food.

Lower-protein foods include bread, fruits, vegetables, pasta, and rice. Low-sodium foods include fresh and frozen vegetables (without sauces), such as greens, broccoli, cauliflower, and peppers; fresh, frozen or dried fruits, such as berries, apples, bananas, and pears; and grains and beans, such as dried beans, brown rice, farro, quinoa, and whole-wheat pasta. Lower-potassium foods include fruits, such as apples, cranberries, grapes, pineapples, and strawberries; vegetables, such as cauliflower, onions, peppers, radishes, summer squash, and lettuce; breads, such as pita, tortillas, and white breads; and proteins, such as beef and chicken. And lower-phosphorous foods include Italian, French, or sourdough bread; corn or rice cereals and cream of wheat; unsalted popcorn; and some light-colored sodas and lemonade.

As the kidney disease worsens, you should decrease the amount of your daily fluid intake. That's to compensate for the loss of kidney function to remove fluids from the body. Fluid retention could lead to swelling in your arms and legs, high blood pressure, or fluid in your lungs (pulmonary edema).

You still need to stay hydrated during exercise. Use the urine color test to make sure you have consumed enough fluid.

Fueling Plates for Kidney Disease

Good portion control is an important part of any meal plan. It is even more important in a kidney-friendly meal plan because you may need to limit how much of certain things you eat and drink. If you are a kidney disease patient, you need to make adjustments to the Healthy Plate. Have a thorough discussion with your nephrologist (kidney specialist) about how much protein and carbohydrates you should have at every meal. There are too many individual factors involved for us to give you specific food recommendations. Talk with your kidney specialist about what you can and can't eat. This is one case that the Healthy Plate needs to be adjusted individually with information exchanged between you and your doctor.

CONCLUSION

My *patients,* and those who have heard my talks about exercise nutrition all across the world, consider me a partner in getting themselves on the path to better eating and drinking. Learning how to properly fuel their body through the lens of a sports-medicine professional, and taking into account their needs as active people, has whipped them into the best shape of their lives. Average people can enhance their everyday activities, too, with the Fueling Plates program.

I became a doctor in order to help people, and I'm proud to have assisted everyone from professional athletes to everyday people. As I've done so, I've found that equally as important as keeping one's muscles, bones, joints and ligaments healthy is paying attention to what you're putting in your body. I'm excited to finally offer a book that answers the questions my patients have been asking me for years. Now you can spend less time trying to distinguish between fact and fallacy, and build a simple, individualized nutritional program that will help you spend more time exercising and doing what you love.

PART FOUR

Celebrity Chef Recipes

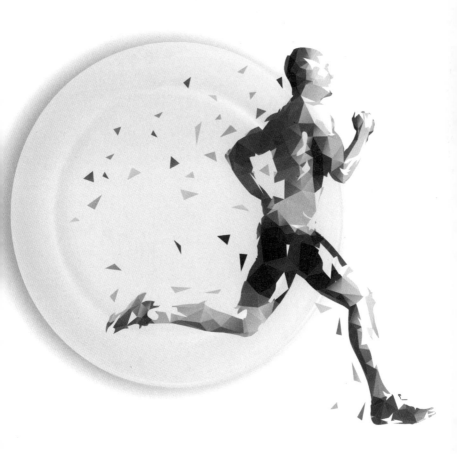

J ust as professional athletes have sought my nutrition advice over the years, so celebrity chefs have knocked on my door when they're looking to get into shape—and now they are here to help you. I have obtained recipes from high-profile chefs from restaurants I frequent in Manhattan, including Craft and Sardi's, and also from culinary innovator Peter Callahan. After each recipe, I give you my notes on where to find the protein, carbohydrates, and fats in each dish. Using the Fueling Plates, you just put the appropriate amount into sections of your plate, and enjoy!

The Craft chefs have designed four recipes, one for each of the four Fueling Plates. The other chefs provided their recipes for you to practice moving food around on your plate. Have fun with these!

CRAFT

New York City restaurant Craft, a James Beard Award-winner with three stars from the *New York Times*, has altered the landscape of fine dining in America by highlighting pristine, seasonal ingredients with simply prepared, family-style dishes and warm hospitality. The restaurant mimics the experience of dining in someone's home—simply prepared dishes with seasonal ingredients served family-style.

I've always found the food at Craft very healthy and fresh. They go by the mantra the more color, the fresher the vegetable. The farm-to-table style of food is served with simple recipes. In fact, the restaurant lists all the farms they receive food from, so you know it's fresh.

The following recipes from Craft highlight the freshness of the ingredients, and that makes it easier to separate out the food into a Fueling Plate.

HEALTHY PLATE

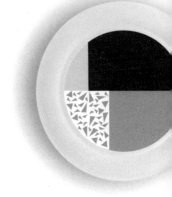

Seared Tuna Bowl with Quinoa, Spinach, Roasted Asparagus, and Champagne Vinaigrette

Yield: 1 serving

Tuna

INGREDIENTS:

6 ounces yellowfin tuna

Salt and pepper to taste

1 teaspoon olive oil

PREPARATION:

Season both sides of tuna with salt and pepper. Place oil in hot skillet and sear tuna on both sides, about 3 minutes each side. Remove from heat and allow to rest. Slice on the diagonal.

Quinoa

INGREDIENTS:

1 cup quinoa

1¾ cup water

1 teaspoon salt

PREPARATION:

Rinse quinoa thoroughly with cold water, drain with a fine mesh strainer. Allow to dry for about 20 minutes. Place quinoa in a dry pan and toast until it gives off a nutty aroma (about 5 to 10 minutes), then remove from heat. In a separate saucepan, boil 1¾ cups of water, then add toasted quinoa to boiling water. Cover with slight vent. Reduce heat to a strong simmer for about 15 to 20 minutes until water is all gone. Remove lid and allow to cool 10 minutes. Fluff with a fork and set aside.

Champagne Vinaigrette

INGREDIENTS:

¼ cup Champagne vinegar	½ tablespoon Dijon mustard
2 tablespoons agave nectar	½ cup olive oil
1 tablespoon fresh lemon juice	Salt and pepper to taste

PREPARATION:

Place vinegar, agave nectar, lemon juice and mustard in a blender and pulse to combine.

With motor running slowly, add oil in a steady stream. Blend until creamy. Season to taste with salt and pepper.

Roasted Asparagus

INGREDIENTS:

1 bunch asparagus	Salt and pepper to taste
1 teaspoon extra virgin olive oil	1 cup baby spinach

PREPARATION:

Remove woody stalk of asparagus (about 2 to 3" from bottom). Cut asparagus into thirds and toss with 1 teaspoon of olive oil, and season to taste with salt and pepper. Place on a sheet lined with aluminum foil (make sure asparagus is spread out). Broil on high for about 10 to 15 minutes until asparagus is slightly charred.

Assemble dish in a bowl: add ½ cup of cooked quinoa, ½ cup of roasted asparagus, and 1 cup of baby spinach. Drizzle vinaigrette over the bowl and then top with sliced seared tuna.

Running Doc note:

If I ordered this dish in the restaurant, I would ask for an extra plate and separate out the ingredients, not mix them together into a bowl. This is an example of a chef not liking me when I deconstruct the beautiful presentation.

The tuna is your protein; quinoa, asparagus, and spinach are slow-acting carbohydrates. You want champagne vinaigrette on the side because that's the fat. I would add in an order of mashed potatoes for some fast-acting carbohydrates.

These ingredients are very healthy. The quality of ingredients helps. At home, if you substituted canned tuna fish from the supermarket for the fresh tuna, it would make a huge difference in flavor and nutrients. Obviously, the fresh fish is better. As for the asparagus, the greener, the better. Also, if you oversteam or boil asparagus, instead of roasting them, they tend to get mushy and you lose some of the valuable micronutrients. Cook asparagus al dente, with bright greenness, for the most nutrients.

TRAINING PLATE

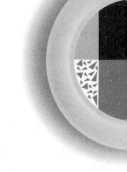

Blackened Red Snapper with Broccoli and Black-Eyed Peas with Brown Rice

Yield: 1 serving

Blackening Seasoning

INGREDIENTS:

2 tablespoons smoked paprika

1 tablespoon brown sugar

1 tablespoon dried oregano

1 tablespoon dried thyme

½ teaspoon cayenne
  (depending on your spice level)

1 teaspoon onion powder

1 teaspoon fresh black pepper

1 teaspoon garlic powder

1 teaspoon salt

PREPARATION:

Mix all ingredients in a bowl. Reserve the rest for future use.

Blackened Red Snapper

INGREDIENTS:

6 ounces fillet of red snapper

½ lemon

Blackening seasoning

PREPARATION:

Liberally coat fillet with blackening seasoning. Place red snapper on sheet tray lined with foil. Broil on high for 10 minutes. Remove from oven; squeeze lemon over fish.

Black-Eyed Peas with Brown Rice

INGREDIENTS:

½ yellow onion, chopped

2 cloves garlic, minced

1 celery stalk, diced

Black pepper to taste

¾ cup water

2 cups cooked brown rice

1½ cups black-eyed peas

½ red bell pepper, stemmed, seeded, and chopped

½ teaspoon hot sauce

PREPARATION:

In a large pan, lightly sauté onion, garlic, celery, and black pepper. Add water and bring to a boil, then add black-eyed peas. Return to boil, stirring frequently. Reduce heat to low, cover, and simmer about 15 minutes until most of the water has evaporated. Add rice and bell pepper and stir. Season to taste.

Roasted Broccoli

INGREDIENTS:

1 head broccoli, cut into florets

1 teaspoon extra virgin olive oil

Salt and pepper to taste

PREPARATION:

Preheat oven to broil. Place broccoli on a sheet tray lined with foil. Pour olive oil on broccoli. Broil on high about 5 to 10 minutes until broccoli is charred.

Serve one fish fillet with 1 cup of broccoli and 1½ cups of black-eyed peas and rice mixture.

Running Doc note:

Red snapper is a healthy protein with fish oils; the black-eyed peas and brown rice mixture and the broccoli are slow-acting carbohydrates. There is a little fat from the olive oil on the broccoli, but you could add a pat of butter to the rice mixture for more fat. I would also add a handful of cherry tomatoes for fast-acting carbohydrates. You need some fast-acting carbohydrates to build up glycogen needed for training.

If you don't like red snapper, it's easy to get fillet of flounder or sole from your local fish shop. Or you could use the same recipe with a lobster tail or scallops.

NIGHT-BEFORE-AN-EVENT PLATE

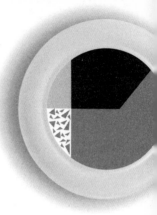

Chicken Breast with Farro Salad

Yield: 1 serving

Chicken

INGREDIENTS:

6 ounces skinless chicken breast

1 teaspoon extra virgin olive oil

Salt and pepper to taste

PREPARATION:

In a hot skillet place the olive oil and the chicken breast, cook 5 minutes on both sides or until internal temperature is 165°F.

Farro Salad

INGREDIENTS:

1 cup farro

4 cups water

1 cup string beans

1 cup heirloom cherry tomatoes, cut in half

2 cups baby arugula

1½ tablespoons extra virgin olive oil

½ lemon

Salt and pepper to taste

PREPARATION:

Bring 4 cups of salted water to boil and add farro. Strain when farro berries have burst, but are still *al dente*, about 25 minutes (cook like pasta). Place cooked farro on sheet tray and allow to cool at room temperature. Trim ends off string beans and cut in half. Blanch string beans in boiling water for about 4 minutes. Remove from boiling water and place in ice water bath. Once cooled remove string beans from water and pat dry.

In large bowl, add farro, string beans, tomatoes, arugula, juice of ½ a lemon, olive oil, and salt and pepper to taste. Toss all ingredients together.

Serve 1½ cups of salad with sliced chicken breast.

Running Doc note:

Chicken breast is the protein in this dish, farro and string beans are slow-acting carbohydrates, and tomatoes are fast-acting carbohydrates. The olive oil provides fat.

Chicken is a low-fat protein, which makes it perfect just before a long event. The night before an event, you need to eat protein so your body can use the amino acids after the event to help build back muscle fibers. Chicken is better than meatballs, which usually have a high fat content and move slowly through the gut during exercise.

AFTER-A-LONG-WORKOUT PLATE

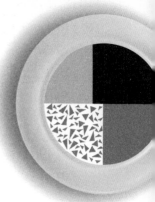

Roasted Pork Loin with Braised Kale and Cannellini Beans

Yield: 1 serving

Roast Pork Loin

INGREDIENTS:

- 1 pork loin at room temperature
  (about 30 minutes out of fridge)
- 3 tablespoons extra virgin olive oil
- 4 garlic cloves, minced
- 1 teaspoon salt
- 1 teaspoon black pepper
- 1 teaspoon fresh sage, chopped
- 1 teaspoon fresh rosemary, chopped
- 2 teaspoons fresh thyme, chopped

PREPARATION:

Preheat oven to 350°F. In a bowl, mix all ingredients except pork loin. Coat pork loin with mixture and place in roasting pan. Roast pork until reaching internal temperature of 145°F (about 30 to 40 minutes). Remove from oven and loosely tent with foil and rest for 15 minutes. Slice thinly.

Braised Beans and Kale ─────────────

INGREDIENTS:

2 tablespoons extra virgin olive oil

1 cup yellow onion, chopped

6 cloves garlic, minced

2 tablespoons fresh thyme, chopped

1 teaspoon tomato paste

1 bunch kale, destemmed and
chopped

1 cup unsalted chicken stock

2 teaspoons lemon zest

2 15-ounce cans cannellini
beans, rinsed and drained

1 15-ounce can diced tomatoes

Parmesan cheese, grated

Salt and pepper to taste

PREPARATION:

In a sauté pan, add 1 tablespoon olive oil, onion, garlic, and thyme and sauté 5 minutes. Then add tomato paste and sauté 3 minutes. Add kale and cook an additional 5 minutes until kale is wilted. Add chicken stock and remaining ingredients. Simmer 10 minutes, stirring occasionally. Add salt and pepper to taste and simmer an additional 5 minutes.

Serve 1½ cups of braised beans and kale topped with 8 ounces of pork loin. Drizzle with olive oil and a little Parmesan cheese.

Running Doc note:

Roast pork, the new white meat, is the protein. It is high in protein and low in fat, much less fat than steak. The beans and kale provide slow-acting carbohydrates, tomatoes are the fast-acting carbohydrates, and the little amount of fat comes from the olive oil.

After a long event or workout, you need to refuel your body. The slow-acting carbohydrates replenish glycogen stores, and fast-acting carbohydrates give you more active energy. These carbohydrates help you reload the energy you expended and repair microtears in muscles.

SARDI'S

Ever since I was a four-year-old boy going to Broadway shows, I went to Sardi's restaurant, and still do for the delicious food. The Broadway theatre would never have been the same without Sardi's. Plays have been written and entirely financed at Sardi's, and hit shows have celebrated their opening at Sardi's. To hang your drawing on the wall at Sardi's is to make your mark on the history of the American stage.

Shrimp Sardi

Yield: 4 servings

INGREDIENTS:

- 2 pounds medium shrimp *(16 to 20)*, peeled *(save shells)*
- 1 small carrot, chopped
- 4 garlic cloves, finely chopped
- 1 stalk of celery, chopped
- 1 white onion, chopped
- 1 large tomato, cubed
- 1 cup white wine
- 1½ cups fish stock or chicken stock
- 1 branch thyme
- ½ bay leaf
- 3 stems parsley
- 3 stems tarragon
- 1½ ounces olive oil
- 3 ounces butter
- 2 teaspoons tomato puree
- 1 French baguette or Italian bread loaf

Sauce

PREPARATION:

In a medium-sized pot, put a few drops of olive oil, add chopped vegetables (do not add the tomato), and cook until colored lightly. Add the shrimp shells (color will change to a reddish color), add white wine, let reduce by half. Then add fish or chicken stock and all herbs, spoon in tomato puree and the cubed tomato. Simmer for 20 minutes on a very low flame. Strain. Keep the juice on the oven until it has a strong shrimp flavor. Remove from flame and whisk in butter. Season to taste. (To make spicy, add ground cayenne pepper.)

Shrimp

PREPARATION:

In a very hot frying pan add olive oil, when hot, add the shrimp, which has been seasoned lightly with salt and pepper. Sauté over low heat (do not overcook). Shrimp will turn a pinkish-red color. One minute prior to removing from flame, add 1 teaspoon of finely chopped garlic, then add the sauce. Do not boil.

PRESENTATION:

In the center of the plate place two croutons made from French or Italian bread. Place the shrimp around the croutons. Pour the sauce to cover all the food. Sprinkle with chopped tarragon or chives. Serve with white rice.

Running Doc note:

This is an iconic Sardi's dish. Shrimp is a good source of protein. The chef suggests white rice as a carbohydrate, but you can use whatever rice appeals to you. White rice is more of a fast-acting carbohydrate; brown or basmati rice are more slow-acting carbohydrates. Personally, I like to eat this dish with a non-starchy vegetable, such as carrots or broccoli, both slow-acting carbohydrates.

You can cut down on the amount of butter, if you like, but don't be too concerned about the fats, particularly after a long workout or event. The After-a-Long-Workout Plate allows for more fats. You already know by now that butter is a fat, and olive oil is a healthier fat.

How much sauce you decide to eat is up to you. The carrot, onion, and tomato in the sauce make it healthier and tastier. When you eat good-tasting entrees and put them into appropriate sections of Fueling Plates, it makes the dish healthy.

Even though the chef has provided a presentation, you are going to move food around on the plate to match your Fueling Plate.

Braised Osso Bucco en Casserole

Yield: 6 servings

INGREDIENTS:

6 veal knuckles

¾ cup shortening

2 onions, chopped

1 carrot, chopped

3 stalks celery, diced

4 teaspoons rosemary

½ teaspoon pepper

1 teaspoon salt

4 cloves garlic, chopped

1 bay leaf

2 cups white wine

2 cups canned tomatoes

2 cups tomato purée

1 tablespoon roux *(made from equal parts flour and fat)*

3 cups white rice

PREPARATION:

Brown knuckles in shortening. When thoroughly browned, take out of the frying pan and place in a pot. Add onions, carrots, and celery to fat in frying pan and brown, stirring well for about 10 minutes. Strain fat off vegetables and place with the meat. To this add rosemary, pepper, salt, garlic, bay leaf, and wine. Cool. Place in refrigerator to marinate for at least 4 hours, or overnight if possible. Next day or later the same day, take out of refrigerator, add tomatoes and tomato purée and bring to a boil. Cover and continue cooking for about 1 hour. Remove from the fire and carefully take out veal knuckles. Place in bowl, cover, and keep warm. Strain the sauce through cheesecloth or fine sieve and return to the fire. Simmer the sauce for 30 minutes. Skim from time to time. If the sauce is a little strong, add some chicken broth. At this time, also add 1 tablespoon roux so that sauce will coat the meat. Cook for 10 minutes. Season to taste and strain once more, this time through a metal strainer only.

Mix white rice with 6 cups of water and cook for 20 minutes or until all water is absorbed. Remove from heat for 5 minutes.

Serve one knuckle of osso bucco over rice to each person.

Running Doc note:

Veal knuckles as a protein are fairly lean since the fat cooks off the meat. Vegetables in the recipe add taste. The chef recommends white rice, which is a fast-acting carbohydrate. I like to have a vegetable side dish to fill me up, such as carrots, broccoli, or asparagus, and to provide slow-acting carbohydrates. When you use wine in this recipe, choose a quality wine, like a chardonnay, instead of cooking wine from the supermarket, for better flavor.

The chef recommends one knuckle per person. You may need more than one knuckle to reach the appropriate protein amount for your Fueling Plate. I would move the rice and vegetables into the section of the plate for carbohydrates and the veal knuckle into the protein part of the plate.

I went to dinner with four professional runners at Sardi's. One runner from South Africa said one of his favorite dishes was osso bucco, but he thought it was unhealthy. I explained he could use the Fueling Plate system to make it healthy. I ordered it and separated out the dish, making an unhealthy-appearing dish into a healthy one. Afterward, he asked the waiter to take back his salmon and bring him an osso bucco, too!

Pan-Roasted Canadian Salmon with Black Bean Sauce

Yield: 4 servings

INGREDIENTS:

Fillet of salmon, skinless and boneless, cut in 4 pieces of 6 ounces each

Salt and pepper

½ teaspoon sesame oil mixed with 1 teaspoon corn oil

3 teaspoons Chinese black beans or fermented black beans

2 large cloves garlic, coarsely chopped

1 walnut-size piece of fresh ginger, cut in fine julienne

Dry white wine, ½ bottle *(750 milliliters)*

2 tablespoons sugar

Dry sherry wine, 2 tablespoons

3 tablespoons low sodium soya sauce

1 tablespoon cornstarch, dissolved in 1 tablespoon water

4 scallions, cut finely on the diagonal

1 large pinch fresh cilantro leaves

1 small pinch red chili flakes, if you desire a little spicy flavor *(optional)*

PREPARATION:

Preheat oven to 350°F. Lightly season the salmon with salt and pepper, then sauté briefly with sesame oil and corn oil (mixed 50/50) in a very hot frying pan for 2 minutes on each side or until nicely colored. Set aside. Rinse the black beans with cool water, drain, and chop coarsely. In a saucepan, sauté the garlic with a little sesame/corn oil, add ginger, white wine, and sugar, bring to a boil. Then simmer gently until reduced by half and add the dry sherry and the black beans. Simmer another few minutes, add the soya sauce, and simmer again for one minute. Then add the cornstarch and taste for seasoning. Place the salmon in a large platter enough to hold it flat, pour the sauce on top, place it in the hot oven, and cook it to your liking. When you remove the salmon from the oven, sprinkle with scallions and cilantro.

Chef's Note:

It's suggested to cook the salmon medium rare. You may serve this dish with stir-fried spinach, jasmine rice, and diced red bell pepper stir fried with garlic and fresh cilantro.

Running Doc note:

Salmon is a protein with a high amount of healthy fish oils. Black beans are a great source of slower-acting carbohydrates. The chef suggests jasmine rice, which is a middle-type carbohydrate, and stir-fried spinach, which is a slow-acting carbohydrate. If you want a fast-acting carbohydrate, use short-grain white rice or mashed pumpkin. The small amount of sugar and low-sodium soya sauce in this dish limit the amount of sugar and salt. I prefer not to oversalt this dish, but you can add salt to taste.

Pan-Roasted Pork Tenderloin "Wild Boar Style"

Yield: 4 servings

INGREDIENTS:

4 pieces pork tenderloin, cut to 7 ounces each	3 cups low-sodium chicken stock
2 pounds pork bone, cut small	Black peppercorns
2 carrots, peeled and sliced	1 celery stalk, sliced
2 Spanish onions, sliced	1.5-liter bottle merlot or cabernet wine
1 head garlic, peeled and cut in half	Cognac
2 bay leaves	3 ounces butter
1 bunch parsley	2 teaspoons flour
2 branches thyme	2 tablespoons olive oil

Marinade

PREPARATION:

One day before, make the marinade. Take half of the vegetables and add to a hot frying pan with 4 teaspoons olive oil. Sauté until nicely colored, then strain the excess oil. Pour in half of the red wine; let it simmer until the vegetables are lightly cooked. Remove from the fire and let it completely cool off.

Note: It is very important that the wine and vegetables are very cold.

Take a deep dish, deep enough to contain the meat, then cover the meat with the marinade (wine and vegetables). Add 1 bay leaf, 1 thyme branch, 10 black peppercorns, and drizzle with a little olive oil. Then place dish in the refrigerator for up to 24 hours. Turn the meat over several times.

Note: Please ask your butcher to cut the two pounds of pork bones in small pieces, in order to make the brown pork broth.

Brown Pork Broth

PREPARATION:

Set oven to 375°F. Put pork bones in a large roasting pan and place the pan in the oven. Let the pork bones color and then add the rest of the vegetables until colored. Remove from the oven and remove the excess fat. Place in a stockpot, add a teaspoon of flour, cook until lightly brown, and add the rest of the red wine, the low-sodium chicken stock, 1 bay leaf, 1 branch of thyme, and the bunch of parsley. Bring to a boil and then simmer very slowly for 2 hours (skimming any fat). At completion, strain the pork stock in another smaller pot; reduce the stock until you get approximately 2 cups of sauce.

The day of serving, lift the tenderloin out of the marinade, pick out any bits of the vegetables and pat the meat dry with a kitchen towel. Strain the marinade through a China cap in a skillet. Reduce on low heat, until you are left with a few tablespoons. Keep on the side.

Finishing the sauce. Crack 15 black peppercorns, sauté in a frying pan, then add 2 good spoonfuls of cognac. For flambé, add the peppercorns to the brown pork sauce, and then add the marinade reduction. Place it on low heat and simmer for a few minutes until the sauce is thick enough to cover the meat (but not too thick). Then season the meat with salt and pepper to taste. It must be a little peppery. Then add butter (do not boil anymore).

Cooking the pork tenderloin. Set oven to 375°F. Choose a skillet that can accommodate the 4 pieces of pork tenderloin without overlapping. Put in one tablespoon olive oil and a little butter, and turn the heat to high. When the oil-butter mixture begins to sizzle, put in the meat, and brown evenly all around. Place the skillet in the oven after 10 minutes, turn the meat over and cook the other side for another 10 minutes. Transfer the meat to a cutting board, cut it into ¼-inch thick slices, then place on a very warm platter or plate and pour the sauce on top.

Serve with roasted root vegetables, mashed potatoes, wild mushrooms, or seasonal vegetables.

Running Doc note:

When I look at the diners at Sardi's, it seems that one out of eight people order this recipe, which is becoming a new standard. Pork is a healthy protein. Wild Boar style means the deep flavor has a mild gamey taste. With the brown pork broth, I suggest you get some good bread to dip in it because it's so delicious, like comfort food.

The chef suggests serving it with roasted root vegetables, mashed potatoes, wild mushrooms, or seasonal vegetables—a good mix of slow-acting carbohydrates (root vegetables, wild mushrooms, and seasonal vegetables), and fast-acting carbohydrates (mashed potatoes). I find this gravy is so delicious with mashed potatoes.

The low-sodium chicken stock is not too salty. Most restaurants make their own chicken stock. If you cook this at home, take the time to make your own chicken stock, too. Boil a whole chicken with root vegetables in water for a few hours and then strain it. Chicken stock from the supermarket has too much sodium and changes the whole taste of the dish. You are better off using salt and pepper to taste with homemade chicken stock.

When you make this dish at home, instead of pouring the sauce directly on the meat, put it on one portion of your plate and dip the meat into it.

Boccone Dolce ("Sweet Bite")

Yield: 8 servings

INGREDIENTS:

4 egg whites

Salt

¼ teaspoon cream of tartar

1 cup sugar

6 ounces semi-sweet chocolate
pieces

3 tablespoons water

3 cups heavy cream

⅓ cup confectioners' sugar

A few drops vanilla extract

1 pint fresh strawberries, sliced

Meringue Layers

PREPARATION:

Preheat oven to 250°F. Beat until stiff 4 egg whites, pinch of salt, and ¼ teaspoon cream of tartar. Gradually beat in 1 cup sugar and continue to beat until the meringue is stiff and glossy. Line baking sheets with wax paper, on the paper trace 3 circles, each 8 inches in diameter. Spread the meringue evenly over the circles, about ½-inch thick, and bake for 20 to 25 minutes or until the meringue is pale gold but still pliable. Remove from oven and carefully peel wax paper from bottom. Put on cake rack to dry.

Filling

PREPARATION:

Melt over hot water 6 ounces semi-sweet chocolate pieces and 3 tablespoons water.

Whip 3 cups heavy cream until stiff. Gradually add ⅓ cup confectioners' sugar and a few drops of vanilla extract and beat until very stiff.

PRESENTATION:

Place a meringue layer on serving plate and spread with a thin covering of melted chocolate. Spread a layer about ¾-inch thick of whipped cream and top with a layer of strawberries, then put on third layer of meringue. Frost sides smoothly with remaining whipped cream. Decorate top meringue layer in an informal pattern, using remaining melted chocolate squeezed through a pastry cone with a tiny round opening. Alternatively, you may decorate with whole ripe strawberries. Refrigerate for two hours prior to serving.

Running Doc note:

If you have been using the Fueling Plates program and eating a healthy diet, and you want to give yourself a treat, this is a world-famous dessert that's only available at Sardi's. It has light texture and flavor and a lot of fast-acting carbohydrates. The day after a long event or workout, when you have used up your carbohydrate stores, may be a good time to try this dish. It will taste even better because you are craving sugar from having depleted all your body's glycogen. It's a great way to finish the night and celebrate all of your hard training.

PETER CALLAHAN

Peter Callahan, owner and Creative Director of New York City-based Peter Callahan Catering, is widely credited with having created the mega trend of miniaturized savory and dessert comfort food hors d'oeuvres. He has been a caterer, food stylist, and culinary innovator for more than twenty-five years, appears frequently as a guest entertainer on the *Today* show, and has made frequent appearances on *Martha Stewart, Extra, The Fabulous Life*, and more.

Peter Callahan is one of the most impressive chefs and food creators. When my wife turned fifty and I turned sixty, we hosted a party that he catered. My friends still talk about how good the food was! These dinner recipes are fresh, healthy, bold, and tasty. They are simple to understand and work well with the Fueling Plates program. It's very clear what foods are the protein, carbohydrates, and fat. It's also easy to adapt the recipes. Instead of Tagine chicken, make Tagine shrimp. Instead of branzino, you can use flounder, sole, or snapper. Instead of steak, you may substitute a broiled pork chop. So you really have more than just four recipes.

Tagine Chicken and Couscous, with Chickpeas, Olives, and Pomegranate

Yield: 4 servings

INGREDIENTS:

- 4 garlic cloves, peeled
- 1 2-ounce jar tagine spice
- 2 to 3 tablespoons of extra virgin olive oil to make paste, plus 3 tablespoons for pan
- 4 boneless skin-on chicken breasts
- Preserved lemon slices for garnish

PREPARATION:

Place garlic in a small pot, just cover with olive oil, and cook on high heat. Once it boils, turn down to low heat for approximately 15 minutes or until garlic is soft. Strain garlic from oil and reserve the oil. Place garlic in food processor with tagine spice. With the motor running, add the oil in small increments until you have a spreadable paste. Pat the chicken breasts dry with paper towels and place in a baking pan. Smear the tagine-garlic paste over both sides. Cover the pan with plastic wrap and refrigerate overnight. Bring the chicken up to room temperature at least 30 minutes before cooking. When ready to cook, wipe the chicken clean of all paste.

Preheat oven to 350°F. Heat 3 tablespoons olive oil in a heavy-bottomed, oven-proof sauté pan over high heat until almost smoking. Carefully add the chicken, skin side down. Cook until the skin is crispy, then flip and cook for 2 more minutes. Transfer the pan to the oven and roast until the chicken is cooked through, about 20 minutes.

Couscous with Chickpeas, Olives, and Pomegranate ———

INGREDIENTS:

¼ cup extra virgin olive oil, divided

2 cups Israeli couscous

1 quart water

3 tablespoons coarse salt,
   plus more to season

¼ cup pitted, halved Castelvetrano
   olives, or other large green olives

1 cup cooked chickpeas
   *(drained and rinsed, if
   canned)*

¼ cup pomegranate seeds

Freshly ground pepper to taste

PREPARATION:

Preheat oven to 350°F. On a sheet pan, toss the couscous with 2 tablespoons of the olive oil and spread in an even layer. Roast in oven until lightly browned, about 10 minutes. Fill a medium pot with 1 quart of water, add the 3 tablespoons salt and bring to a boil over medium heat. Add the couscous from the pan to the pot and cook until tender, 8 to 10 minutes. Drain the water from the pot, transfer couscous to a large bowl, and toss with remaining 2 tablespoons olive oil. Add the olives, chickpeas, and pomegranate seeds to the couscous and toss to combine. Season with salt and pepper to taste.

To serve, spoon some of the juices from the pan into the bottom of a bowl, add a mound of couscous, and place a piece of chicken on top. Garnish with a slice of preserved lemon.

Running Doc note:

Delicious, moist chicken is the protein in this dish. Couscous provides mostly slow-acting carbohydrates; the chickpeas and olives are slow-acting carbohydrates, too. This low-fat recipe uses olive oil without lots of butter. Peter uses spices to make it tasty instead of butter. When you marinate the chicken overnight, the taste is in the chicken. You may want to add in some fast-acting carbohydrates, such as dried apricots. The pomegranate seeds add healthy antioxidants.

Pan-Seared, Breaded Branzino Topped with Tomato Confit, Sugar Snap Peas, Royal Trumpet Mushrooms, and Pearl Onions

Yield: 4 servings

Branzino

INGREDIENTS:

8 4-ounce branzino fillets

Coarse salt

2 cups panko

½ cup extra virgin olive oil

¼ cup grape-seed oil

PREPARATION:

Preheat oven to 350°F. Line a baking sheet with parchment paper. Place 2 fillets, 1 on top of the other, skin sides together, to make a thicker fillet. Repeat with the remaining fish for 4 thick fillets. Season both sides of the fillets with salt. In a small bowl, mix panko with olive oil to create a slightly damp mixture that will stick to the fish but retain a crumbly texture. Press the panko mixture on the top of each of the fillets.

Heat large sauté pan to high heat, and add grape-seed oil until almost smoking. Reduce to low heat and place the fillets in the pan, crumb side down. Cook the fillets, without moving them, until golden brown, about 2 minutes.

Carefully remove fillets from pan (it will be hot) and place them, crumb side up, on baking sheet. Bake the fillets in the oven until just cooked through, 7 to 8 minutes. Top the fish with about 2 tablespoons of tomato confit.

Tomato Confit

INGREDIENTS:

4 on-the-vine red tomatoes, cored,
seeded, cut in half
Extra virgin olive oil
1 sheet cheesecloth
3 garlic cloves

1 tablespoon coriander seeds
1 tablespoon white
peppercorns
Kitchen twine
Coarse salt to taste

PREPARATION:

Preheat oven to 250°F. Place the tomatoes cut side down in a baking dish just large enough to hold the tomatoes (about an 8-inch baking dish). Add enough olive oil to cover two-thirds of the tomatoes. Make a cheesecloth sachet containing the garlic, coriander, and white peppercorns and tie off with kitchen twine. Submerge the sachet in the oil in the baking dish. Sprinkle the tomatoes generously with coarse salt.

Cover the dish tightly with aluminum foil and bake for approximately 2 hours or until the tomatoes are very soft. Remove the baking dish from the oven and discard the foil. Take the tomatoes out of the foil with a slotted spoon and place the tomatoes on a plate or baking sheet, skin side up. Carefully pull skin away from tomatoes and discard the skin. (Note: You can transfer the tomatoes to a jar or plastic container and refrigerate for up to a week for later use, if need be. This also freezes well.)

Accompaniments

INGREDIENTS:

1 cup peeled white pearl onions
3 to 4 tablespoons extra virgin
olive oil, plus another
2 to 3 tablespoons
Salt and pepper to taste

2 royal trumpet mushrooms
1 shallot peeled and finely
diced
2 cups water
1 pound cleaned sugar snap peas

PREPARATION:

Preheat oven to 350°F. Toss pearl onions in a bowl with enough olive oil to coat, about 3 to 4 tablespoons. Season with salt and pepper. Place onions on a baking sheet and bake for approximately 20 minutes or until golden brown. Place onions in a large bowl.

Cut trumpet mushrooms in half lengthwise and place flat side down, then cut halves in 4 equal strips. Heat enough oil to cover bottom of a medium sauté pan, about 2 to 3 tablespoons. Place mushrooms in pan, flipping occasionally until both sides are golden brown. Season with salt and pepper. Add shallot to pan and toss with mushrooms. Cook together for 30 seconds, then remove mushrooms and shallots from pan and place in the bowl with the onions.

In a medium pot, boil water and add a pinch of salt. Drop sugar snap peas into the pot of boiling water and cook for approximately 3 to 4 minutes. Remove the sugar snap peas with a slotted spoon and place in the bowl with onions and mushrooms. Toss all vegetables together to form a medley.

Serve branzino over a bed of accompaniments and top with tomato confit.

Running Doc note:

Branzino, a flaky fish similar to sole, contains healthy fish oils, is low in fat, and is a good source of protein. Tomato is a middle-acting carbohydrate. The panko in this dish also provide middle-acting carbohydrates. The pearl onions, mushrooms, and snap peas are slower-acting carbohydrates. You could add in rice of your choice as a faster-acting carbohydrate. I suggest mixing the tomato confit into the rice to make it tastier. The two types of oils, extra virgin and grape seed, are healthy and low in fat.

Pan-Seared Filet Mignon with French Green Beans and Garlic Mashed Potatoes

Yield: 4 servings

INGREDIENTS:

- 4 7-ounce filet mignon steaks, trimmed and portioned by your butcher
- Salt and pepper to taste
- ¼ cup duck fat or olive oil
- 2 cups water
- ½ pound French green beans
- 1 head garlic
- 1 tablespoon olive oil
- 2 cups water
- 2 pounds russet potatoes
- 1 cup whole milk
- 4 tablespoons butter

Filet Mignon

PREPARATION:

Preheat oven to 350°F. Heat large skillet to high heat. While pan is heating, season the steaks with salt and pepper. Once pan is hot, add duck fat or olive oil and place meat in pan. Cook steaks until they have a charred, golden-brown crust, approximately 3 to 4 minutes. Turn and repeat on the other side. Remove the steaks from the pan and place them on a baking sheet. Put baking sheet in oven for approximately 8 to 12 minutes. Cook to desired temperature, 135°F for medium rare.

Green Beans

PREPARATION:

In a medium pot, boil water and add a pinch of salt. Place green beans in the pot and submerge them. Cook the green beans for approximately 5 minutes and then take them out of the water with a strainer.

Mashed Potatoes

PREPARATION:

Separate the head of garlic into individual cloves. Toss in 1 tablespoon of olive oil and tightly wrap garlic cloves in small pieces of aluminum foil. Bake garlic cloves at 350°F for 45 minutes. When the garlic cloves have cooled to the touch, squeeze the garlic out of the peels. Mash the roasted garlic with a fork.

In a medium pot, boil water and add a pinch of salt. Peel potatoes and boil in salted water until tender. Force the cooked potatoes through a ricer or mash with a potato masher. Place potatoes in a large bowl. In a separate small pot, add milk and butter and bring to a light boil. Gradually add the milk and butter mixture to the bowl of potatoes along with the garlic and whisk until desired consistency. Season with salt and pepper.

Serve filet mignon with green beans and mashed potatoes.

Running Doc note:

This dish is very easy to divide on a Fueling Plate. The filet mignon is the protein. Mashed potatoes are fast-acting carbohydrates, and green beans are slow-acting carbohydrates. I would choose olive oil over duck fat because it is healthier. If you have had no fat for a few days, you could choose the duck fat for flavor. The same holds true for mashed potatoes. Peter makes it with whole milk; I would use 1 percent milk. Also, you may substitute low-fat margarine for the butter to reduce the amount of fat. The green beans boiled in salted water may need some additional flavor. I might add one pat of butter on the sautéed green beans for taste. The recipe calls for 4 tablespoons of butter, but that's one tablespoon for each of the four servings, so it's not really that much butter.

Duck Magret, Oven-Roasted Green and White Asparagus, Roasted Fingerling Potatoes

Yield: 4 servings

INGREDIENTS:

1 double-breasted duck magret
(*sold in high-end grocery stores such as Citarella, D'Artagnan brand*)

2 cups fingerling potatoes

¼ cup olive oil

Salt and pepper to taste

2 tablespoons chopped chives

2 tablespoons finely chopped shallots

1 bunch large green asparagus

1 bunch large white asparagus

2 cups water

PREPARATION:

Preheat oven to 425°F. Split double breast of duck into 2 single breasts. Score the skin side of the duck with a knife to make small squares on the skin, being careful not to cut into the meat. In a cast-iron pan, lay the duck breast skin side down. Cook on high heat for 8 minutes, then lower to medium heat and cook for 4 more minutes. Let the duck rest for 5 minutes and then slice it into ⅛-inch thick slices.

Toss potatoes in olive oil, sprinkle liberally with salt and pepper, and lay the potatoes flat on a baking sheet. Place in oven for 30 minutes. When done, put potatoes into a large bowl and toss in chives and shallots.

Wash and dry the asparagus and then cut about one inch off the bottom of all asparagus spears. Lightly peel the spears from just below the tip to the bottom. In a medium pot, boil water and add a pinch of salt. Drop asparagus into the pot and cook for approximately 5 minutes or until tender.

Serve duck with asparagus and potatoes.

Running Doc note:

Duck is a fatty bird, but cooking the breast in this way cooks off some of the fat. Scoring the skin side with a knife allows for fat under the skin to cook out and fall into the pan. So this duck meat is actually a healthier protein. The potatoes are fast-acting carbohydrates, and asparagus is slow-acting carbohydrates. You may want to add in a pat of butter on top of the asparagus after they are cooked. Peter uses both white and green asparagus to add color and make it look better on the plate. If food looks good, it probably tastes good. Roasted fingerling potatoes are smaller potatoes with lots of flavor. Chives and shallots (a cross between garlic and onion) also add taste. The duck breast can also be purchased at a butcher shop.

FUELING PLATES DIAGRAMS

Healthy Plate

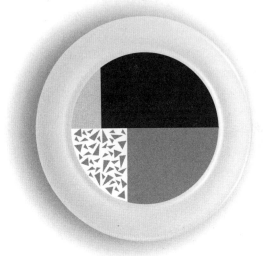

Training Plate

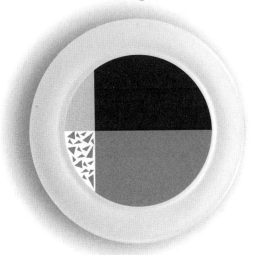

gend: light gray = low fat; black = protein; dark gray = slow-acting carbs; speckled = fast-acting carbs

Night-Before-an-Event Plate

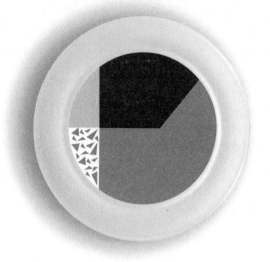

After-a-Long-Workout Plate

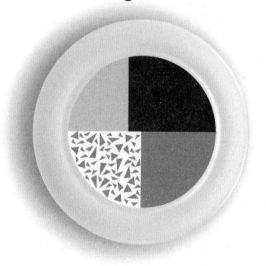

Legend: light gray = low fat; black = protein; dark gray = slow-acting carbs; speckled = fast-acting car

INDEX

Note: *c* after a page number indicates a chart; *d*, a diagram.

A

Acetylcholine and ketone production, 13
Active transport pump, 35
Adenosine triphosphate (ATP) production, 12–13, 59–60
Adolescent sports nutrition, 184–185
Advertising as eating behavior influence, 103
Aerobic exercise, 107, 141–142, 145, 155, 158, 161, 194–196
After-a-Long-Workout Plate, 123–129, 125*d*, 252*d*
    beer, 129
    energy restoration, 125–126
    glycogen replenishment, 125
    low-fat chocolate milk, 128–129
    massage, 127
    post-event soreness reduction, 126
    protein to build muscles provision, 126
    recovery and nutritional needs, 124
    rehydration, 126
    timing, 127–128
Age and cholesterol, 47
Alcohol and HDL, 54
Alpha-linolenic acid and vegetarian Healthy
        Plate, 100
Amenorrhea, 173–174
Amino acid conversion, 13
Anabolic steroids, 64–74
    androstenedione and DHEA, 70–72
    corticosteroids compared, 64–65
    creatine, 72–74
    dangers, 65
    effects, 66
    females and, 69–70
    history, 65
    pyramiding, 67

    regulation, 66
    side effects, 67–69
    stacking, 67
    testosterone, 66
    uses, 65
Androstenedione and DHEA, 70–72
Anemia, 170
Anorexia, 172, 190
Antioxidants, 22–25
    excess antioxidants, health risk of, 23
    free radicals, 22
    oxidative stress, 23
    sources, 24–25
Athlete's heart, 195–196
ATP production. *See* Adenosine triphosphate
        (ATP) production

B

Bad fats, 14–15
    effects of, 14–15
    saturated fats, 14
    sources, 15
    trans fats, 14
Baseball and softball nutrition, 150–151
Basketball nutrition, 151
BCAA. *See* Branched chain amino acids (BCAA)
Beans as superfood, 20
Beer and After-a-Long Workout Plate, 129
Blackened Red Snapper with Broccoli and Black-
        Eyed Peas with Brown Rice Training
        Plate, 218–220
Blood sugar testing for diabetes, 203–204
Blueberries as superfood, 19–20
Boccone Dolce ("Sweet Bite"), 235–236
Body image and teens, 189–190
    anorexia, 190
    fat talk, 189–190
Bone density, 171

ABOUT THE AUTHOR

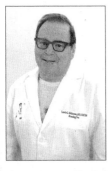

Lewis G. Maharam, MD, FACSM, is one of the world's most extensively credentialed and well-known sports medicine and running health experts. Better known as Running Doc,™ he has been a primary-care sports-medicine physician for more than three decades and currently runs a private practice in New York City. Maharam is the past medical director of the Rock 'n' Roll Marathon series and current medical director of the Leukemia & Lymphoma Society's Team in Training Program and former medical director of the New York Road Runners Club and the New York City Marathon. He has appeared on *World News Tonight, Today, Good Morning America, Inside Edition,* CNN, and Fox News.

Dr. Maharam is chairman of the International Marathon Medical Directors Association and a member of the American College of Sports Medicine's Public Information Committee. He is former president of the Greater New York Chapter of ACSM. He was appointed Team USA physician in track and field for the 1999 World Indoor Championships in Japan. He served previously as the team physician for the Team USA junior track and field team that won the IAAF Championship in Sydney in 1996.

Dr. Maharam graduated from Atlanta's Emory University School of Medicine. Internships and residencies followed at Columbia Presbyterian Hospital and Yale Hospitals prior to a fellowship with Dr. Allan Levy, the team physician with the New York Giants, in primary care sports medicine, where he also gleaned information from Giants' team nutritionists. Following this, he entered private practice, where his unique credentials led him to the Mount Sinai School of Medicine as both an adjunct assistant professor in orthopaedic surgery and an adjunct assistant professor in internal medicine.

Dr. Maharam has written for *Runner's World* and *Competitor* magazines and authored the books *Maharam's Curve: The Exercise High— How to Get it, How to Keep It; Backs in Motion,* which was published in paperback as *A Healthy Back;* and *Running Doc's Guide to Healthy Running.*

Mark L. Fuerst is an award-winning health and medical writer and the coauthor of twelve books, including three books on sports injuries with the New York Giants team physician Allan Levy, MD, who was one of Dr. Maharam's mentors. He first met Dr. Maharam at a sports nutrition conference twenty-five years ago. As a freelance journalist for forty years, his articles have appeared in popular consumer magazines such as *Family Circle, Good Housekeeping, Health, Parents, Self, Woman's Day,* and *Woman's World.*

Mr. Fuerst earned a biology degree from Dickinson College and a master's degree in journalism from the University of Missouri at Columbia. He has been a member of the American Society of Journalists and Authors for nearly forty years, for which he served as president from 1992 to 1994. He lives in Brooklyn, New York, with his wife and two children.